Vascular CT
Angiography Manual

Robert Pelberg · Wojciech Mazur

Vascular CT
Angiography Manual

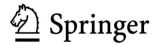 Springer

Authors

Robert A. Pelberg, MD
Ohio Heart and Vascular
Center, The Christ Hospital
Heart and Vascular Center and
The Carl and Edyth Lindner
Center for Research and
Education, 10506 Montgomery
Road Suite 504 Cincinnati,
Ohio 45242
USA

Wojciech Mazur, MD
The Christ Hospital Heart and
Vascular Center and The Carl
and Edyth Lindner Center for
Research and Education
and the Ohio Heart and
Vascular Center,
2123 Auburn Avenue
Cincinnati, Ohio 45219
USA

ISBN 978-1-84996-259-9   e-ISBN 978-1-84996-260-5
DOI 10.1007/978-1-84996-260-5
Springer Dordrecht Heidelberg London New York

Library of Congress Control Number: 2010932884

Cover design: eStudioCalamar Figueres/Berlin

Printed on acid-free paper

Springer is part of Springer Science+Business Media (www.springer.com)

In loving memory of my father, Joe Pelberg and my father-in-law, Jerry Winter.

I would also like to dedicate this book to my loving wife Wendy, my wonderful children, Josh, Adam and Noah, and to my devoted mother, Merryl, my sister Randi, my brother-in-law Michael and my late uncle Merrill Pelberg

Thank you also to Gail Winter and to Miriam, David, Josie and Blake Lieber for their love and support.
Robert Pelberg

To my loving wife and children.
Wojciech Mazur

Foreword

Vision is the Art of Seeing the Invisible
Jonathan Swift
Knowing is not Enough; We Must Apply
Johann Wolfgang Von Goethe

As we lay to rest the first decade of the twenty-first century, we look back at a virtual explosion of diagnostic imaging technology. There is no doubt that computed tomography has led the way.

As a medical resident in the 1980s, I had the good fortune in hind sight, but at that time the dreaded task of sitting with the patients undergoing head CTs in what I thought must have been Sir Godfrey Hounsfield's first commercially available scanner. The initial scanner developed by EMI took 20–30 min to complete 10 slices at 2 slices every 5 min. It was incredibly slow and noisy and what my daughter would call clunky. As the gantry would rotate, it would settle into its next imaging position with a distinct sound of bending metal. The original voxels were in the $3 \times 3 \times 13$ mm range that later were reduced to 1.5×1.5 mm. The neurologist would sit there and glean over the 10 Polaroid-like pictures of the brain that the techs neatly displayed and confer a diagnosis. Jump ahead 30+ years with the introduction of systems that can now acquire 320 images, with a spatial resolution that is submillimeter, and do that in seconds. Work stations that look like my sons' video games and clearly exceed the processing power of the computers used to land a man on the moon, just as Moore's Law would have predicted. The mid-to-late 1990s introduced the ability to take this technology and visualize the coronary tree for the first time noninvasively, bringing cardiologist into the field of CT. To mirror their interventional colleagues, starting with the coronary anatomy both in diagnosis and treatment, and moving into other vascular beds such as carotids, renals, and peripheral run-offs, the imaging cardiologists were asked to look beyond the coronaries.

CT scanning has become the gold standard for evaluating the aorta, from its inception at the heart to its termination at the iliacs, along with all vessels in-between and beyond for aneurysms, dissections, and obstruction. The treatment of vascular disease has also witnessed an amazing evolution, from the advent of endografts for aortic aneurysms to the myriad of specialty devices and stents that are now available for obstructive disease. Today, it is becoming a common place for many of these patients to be evaluated and undergo postinterventional surveillance with CT.

Being able to visualize not only the entire carotid artery, but the arch as well provides the interventionist a unique platform from which to launch his (or her) treatment strategy. Knowing the diameter, length, and take-off trajectory and of any accessory vessels when planning renal artery intervention places CT in the forefront of intervention preparation. Patients with critical limb ischemia have clearly benefited from preintervention CT angiography, being able to decide between catheter-based intervention or surgical revascularization. Planning interventional strategies through imaging in patients who continue to have more and more complex cardiac and vascular disease has made the imaging clinician, both cardiologist and radiologist, an invaluable asset.

As radiation continues to be a "hot-button" topic in the medical imaging arena, we must take a moment to pause. Does the radiation exposure in the CT lab save on radiation in the angiography suite? Is there a significant cancer risk with CTA? Does that risk outweigh or go pale to the risk of cardiac and vascular complications? Many of these strategies will be tested as this field expands.

Pelberg and Mazur's text on Vascular CT Angiography provides an overview from the basic to the esoteric for those of us in the CT and peripheral labs who are confronted with sometimes confounding vascular pathology. I believe this companion will be a highly valuable resource for not only the imaging subspecialists, but also all those taking care of an increasing number of complex vascular patients.

Peter S. Fail, MD, FACC, FACP
Director of the Cardiac Catheterization Laboratories,
Interventional Research and CT Imaging
Cardiovascular Institute of the South

Preface

This book was written for the purpose of making vascular computed tomographic angiography easy and enjoyable. It is the second in our CT angiography series (see *Cardiac CT Angiography Manual*[1]) and is intended to be a useful summary of the field of vascular CT angiography. Once proficient in cardiac CT angiography, training in vascular CT is of greater ease and this book intends to simplify that process. It is not, however, meant to replace formal hands on training.

The information in this work was collected and compiled from peer-reviewed literature, lectures, and textbooks. In addition, we have tried to document the experiences and tips we have learned from the many visiting fellowships and courses we attended. Finally, we have also included information from our experience in performing this technique. We have attempted to be as complete as possible in documenting the sources of our information.

The clinical chapters are all similarly organized. The carotid, thoracic aorta, abdominal aorta, and peripheral vascular chapters contain sections on anatomy, disease states, the accuracy of computed tomography (CT) for each body region, and the approach to reading a CT for each specific anatomical territory. Each chapter is full of helpful figures and wonderful CT image examples.

The field of vascular imaging is ever changing. New research and clinical experience are rapidly advancing vascular medicine and CT angiography is no exception. The authors believe the information in this book to be reliable and in accord with the standards accepted at the time that this document was written. However, in view of the possibility of human error or changes in the field, the authors do not warrant that the information contained herein is in every respect accurate or complete and they are not responsible for any errors or omissions, or for the results obtained from the use of such information. Readers are encouraged to confirm the information herein with other sources. In addition, readers are encouraged to be familiar with the concepts of radiation safety.

Cincinnati Ohio, USA   Robert A. Pelberg
Cincinnati Ohio, USA   Wojciech Mazur

Acknowledgments

A special thanks and appreciation goes to David Collins, a motivated, responsible, and skilled colleague without whom this book would not be possible. In addition, thanks to Tom Kracus from Kettering Medical Center, Dayton Ohio, Russell Hirsch from the University of Cincinnati, Cincinnati, OH and Sanjay Srivatsa from Innovis Health, Fargo, ND who all provided some of the images in this book. Thanks to Chris Telling for his technical expertise in converting our drawings to print format. Many thanks also to Peter Fail from the Cardiovascular Institute of the South in Houma, Louisiana, for his willingness to share his successful imaging protocols and some wonderful cases displayed in this book and for his well written foreword. Finally, thank you to Grant Weston, Cate Rogers and the Springer team for believing in us.

Contents

Chapter 1
Introduction

1.1 Introduction

Atherosclerotic vascular disease is a chronic, progressive disease resulting in narrowing of the arteries supplying blood to the body, excluding the heart. In its most general application, vascular disease would include atherosclerosis of the aorta, the head and neck arteries, the arteries of the upper and lower extremities, the mesenteric arteries, and the renal arteries. Many other disease processes may affect the vascular system and this book will also touch on many of these disease states.

Atherosclerotic vascular disease affects millions of patients in the United States and throughout the world. A systemic process, peripheral atherosclerosis is commonly associated with coronary atherosclerosis and vice versa. Unfortunately, vascular symptoms are present in less than half of those afflicted with this debilitating and potentially life-threatening process and thus it is frequently under-diagnosed and under-treated. Fortunately, if diagnosed in a timely and proper manner, vascular atherosclerosis may be mitigated and the potential morbidity and mortality may be prevented. In addition, with proper vascular screening, other disease processes may be identified and treated as well.

Traditionally, catheter-based angiography was the only accurate method to diagnose vascular illness. However, the twenty-first century has seen the explosion of accurate,

R. Pelberg, W. Mazur, *Vascular CT Angiography Manual*,
DOI: 10.1007/978-1-84996-260-5_1,
© Springer-Verlag London Limited 2011

noninvasive diagnostic tools to assess the body's circulation, including duplex ultrasonography, magnetic resonance imaging, and vascular computed tomographic (CT) angiography.

The earliest CT scanner was developed simultaneously by Sir Godfrey Hounsfield and Allen Cormack, resulting in primitive images of the soft tissue of the brain. Each tomographic slice required hours of scan time and days of post-processing. Over the ensuing decades, scanning speed increased and contrast and spatial resolution improved remarkably. Still though, scanning was relatively slow since each slice was acquired individually while the table was incrementally advanced through an x-ray generator/detector system that was rotated once around the patient for each image.

In the 1990s the slip ring was developed which permitted helical scanning. Here, the x-ray tube/detector array is continuously rotated around the patient as the table is incrementally advanced, resulting in a continuous spiral scanning mechanism through the entire patient. Thus, CT scanning became much more rapid and efficient. The introduction of multiple detector rows allowed further improvement in spatial resolution, and quicker scanning times since fewer slices were required to image a defined field of view. And finally, with advancements in computer technology, large image data sets could be quickly processed and manipulated in real time, thus providing a more complete understanding of the vascular anatomy than traditional invasive angiography since the arterial wall itself may be visualized and the anatomy may be seen from any orientation.

These rapid advancements in CT technology have led to more frequent referrals and earlier treatment of vascular disease. Today, vascular CT angiography is readily available, relatively inexpensive, safe, and accurate. It is now state of the art for the noninvasive diagnosis of vascular illness and for treatment planning techniques and post-treatment surveillance algorithms.

Chapter 2
CT Basics

2.1 Attenuation

Computed tomographic (CT) images are depictions of relative and not absolute tissue densities. These relative depictions are produced by measuring x-ray attenuation resulting from its travel through tissue. A tissue's attenuation is expressed by its attenuation coefficient, μ. μ is an indicator of the likelihood that a photon will interact with an atom of a tissue rather than passing through it. The greater the density of a tissue, the greater its attenuation coefficient. However, specific tissues do not have constant attenuation coefficients. The attenuation coefficient of a tissue is also affected by the photon energy of an x-ray (KeV) and by the tissue thickness. Increasing photon energy and decreasing tissue thickness will reduce the attenuation coefficient of a specific tissue, thus allowing more photons to pass through to the detector (Fig. 2.1).

The CT detector is a photon flux counter where a scintillation detector detects the incident photons and converts them to light. The light is then converted to an electrical signal by the photodiode and the electrical signal is converted to a digital signal by the computer. The photon flux detected by the detector (I) is a function of the photon flux emitted by the x-ray tube (I_0) and the attenuation coefficient (μ) of the tissue where $I = I_0 \times e^{-\mu}$.

As μ increases, the fraction, $e^{-\mu}$, decreases such that the fraction of the incident photons (I_0) detected at the detector (I)

R. Pelberg, W. Mazur, *Vascular CT Angiography Manual*,
DOI: 10.1007/978-1-84996-260-5_2,
© Springer-Verlag London Limited 2011

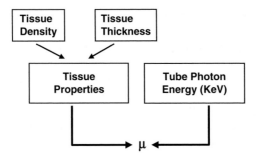

FIGURE 2.1. Figure depicts the factors that influence the attenuation constant μ.

will decrease. The resultant flux at the detector is thus a fraction of the flux emanating from the tube.

2.2 mA Versus KeV

X-ray energy (KeV) represents the energy of each single x-ray emanating from the x-ray tube. The x-ray flux (mA) represents the current or frequency of the x-ray emissions from the x-ray tube. The effect of increasing the KeV is to increase tissue penetration, decrease image noise, increase radiation and decrease tissue contrast. Increasing the mA will decrease the image noise, increase the tissue contrast and increase the radiation dose.

2.3 The Detector and the Calculation of the CT Number

The CT detector counts the x-ray photons that pass through the patient. These detected counts (I) along with the known counts leaving the x-ray detector (I_0) are incorporated into the equation $I = I_0 \times e^{-\mu}$ to calculate the attenuation coefficient (μ). The key point is that the attenuation coefficient (μ) is calculated using count data and not measured directly. From the calculated attenuation coefficient (μ), the CT number is computed using the equation CT number = $[(\mu_{tissue} - \mu_{water})/\mu_{water}] \times 1,000$. The CT number is the Hounsfield unit (HU) number behind the image. As μ increases, less photons reach the detector and, thus, the CT number will increase and the image will brighten. A decreasing μ will result in the opposite effect. The CT number represents the density of the tissue relative to the density of water (Figs. 2.2–2.4).

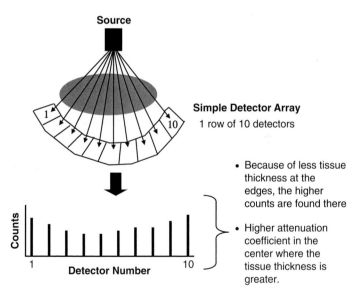

Source

Simple Detector Array
1 row of 10 detectors

- Because of less tissue thickness at the edges, the higher counts are found there

- Higher attenuation coefficient in the center where the tissue thickness is greater.

Counts

Detector Number

FIGURE 2.2. Schematic illustrating the creation of a radiation counts graph as photons are detected by the detector. This is the initial step in creating a computed tomographic (CT) image.

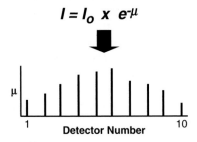

Attenuation Coefficient (μ) is back calculated from the scintillation data using this equation.

$$I = I_o \; x \; e^{-\mu}$$

μ

1   **Detector Number**   10

This graph is opposite the counts graph. Higher counts means lower attenuation coefficient and vice versa. Thus, the μ is lower at the edges and higher in the middle.

FIGURE 2.3. A cartoon illustrating the back calculation of μ from the scintillation data. μ is not measured directly.

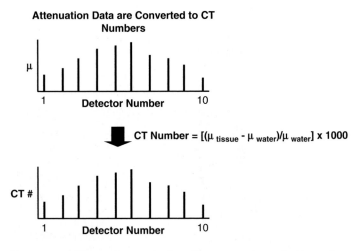

Attenuation Data are Converted to CT Numbers

μ

1   **Detector Number**   10

CT Number = [(μ $_{tissue}$ - μ $_{water}$)/μ $_{water}$] x 1000

CT #

1   **Detector Number**   10

FIGURE 2.4. Figure demonstrating the conversion of attenuation coefficient data to the computed tomographic (CT) numbers using the CT number equation.

2.4 The Matrix

The matrix is the grid of pixels that make up the image. The calculated CT number is projected onto the computer matrix in the location corresponding to the detector location that received the particular incident x-ray photons. The usual matrix size is 512 pixels by 512 pixels because the optimum matrix size is one that most closely matches the pixel size with the inherent spatial resolution of the scanner. If matrix size = displayed field of view (FOV)/pixel size and if the spatial resolution of most scanners is near 0.42 mm and the usual FOV of the heart is 250 mm then the optimum matrix size calculates to 595. Therefore, a 512 by 512 matrix is the best that can be achieved. It is important to note that the matrix size does not have any effect on the spatial resolution (Figs. 2.5 and 2.6).

2.5 Field of View

The FOV is the angular size of the scanned image or the length of the body that is scanned in the Z-axis (head to toe axis). The scanned FOV (sFOV) is the actual longitudinal distance along

CT Number Values are Projected
onto a Matrix Array Based on the
Detector Location

512

512

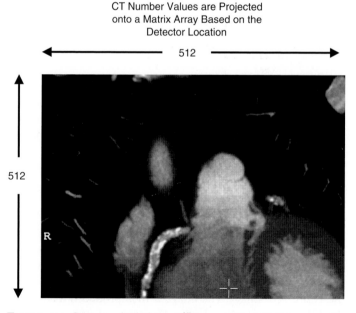

FIGURE 2.5. Cartoon depicting a representation of the computer matrix on which the computed tomographic (CT) image is overlaid. The usual CT matrix size is 512 pixels by 512 pixels.

Each dot represents an individual pixel. The matrix size is 512 pixels by 512 pixels.
Each voxel is the volume of each pixel deep into the screen. By assigning a gray
scale value to each pixel deep into the screen, more shades of gray are possible.
An isotropic voxel is one where the spatial resolution is equal in all 3 planes.
Isotropic voxels are what allow 3-D volume rendered images to be manipulated
without distortion.

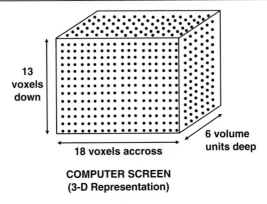

**13
voxels
down**

**6 volume
units deep**

18 voxels accross

**COMPUTER SCREEN
(3-D Representation)**

FIGURE 2.6. Illustration of a computer matrix in cartoon format
(Reproduced with permission from Pelberg R, Mazur W. *Cardiac
CT Angiography Manual.* London: Springer; 2007).

the body that is scanned. The displayed FOV (dFOV) is the portion of the sFOV that is displayed for the reader to review. The
FOV and the matrix size determine the pixel size as noted by
rearranging the formula for matrix size to yield the equation
pixel size = dFOV/matrix size.

2.6 Backprojection

Data from hundreds of projection angles around the gantry
are summed to reconstruct the CT image. Since the data from
a projection of $0°$ is identical to the data from a projection of
$180°$, only a $180°$ gantry rotation is necessary to reconstruct
the entire $360°$ image. The image is then produced from all of
the CT numbers derived from the summed projection data
and from the windowing that is applied to the image on the
screen (Fig. 2.7).

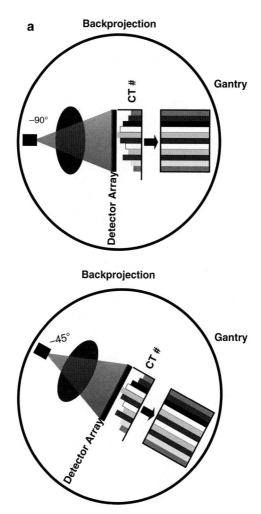

FIGURE 2.7. Cartoon demonstrating the technique of filtered back projection which is used to create the computed tomographic (CT) image. Only a 180° gantry rotation is necessary to encompass a 360° image because the images from 0° and 180° are identical. Hundreds of projection angles are added together to create a CT image. The small, black square represents the x-ray source. The dark grey oval is the patient. The triangle emanating from the x-ray source is the x-ray beam. The final "striped" square is the gantry angle specific back projected image which is added to the other specific back projected images to create the total CT picture.

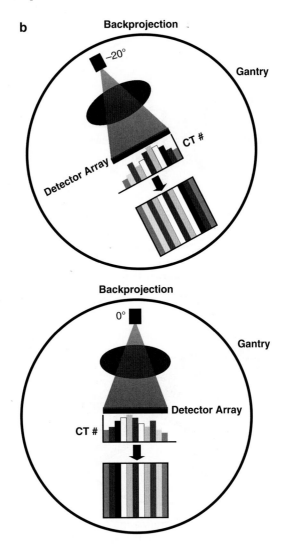

FIGURE 2.7. (continued).

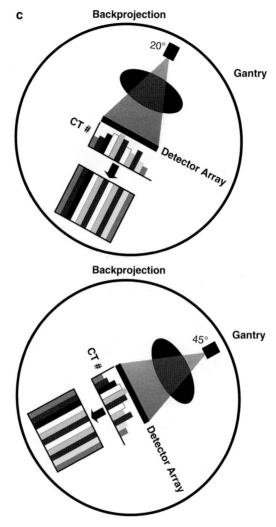

FIGURE 2.7. (continued).

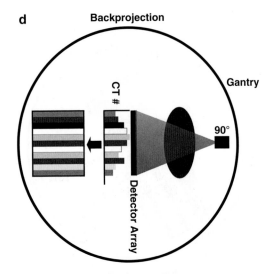

Because the 0 degree and 180 degree projection are identical, only 180 degrees of gantry rotation are necessary to create an image.

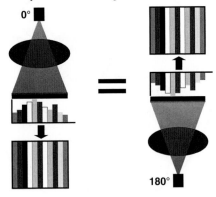

FIGURE 2.7. (continued).

e

CT Image = Matrix of CT # s + Image Window

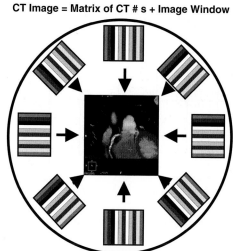

Hundreds of projections are added together to create the CT image.

FIGURE 2.7. (continued).

2.7 Iodine Flux

The iodine flux is the contrast intensity seen in the vessels and vascular chambers. The goal is to have adequate iodine flux in the structures of interest. The many variables that effect the contrast enhancement of a CT image are depicted in Table 2.1.

TABLE 2.1. Effect of many variables on contrast enhancement.

Variable	Contrast enhancement
Increase patient weight	Decrease
Increase patient height	Decrease
Increase Body Mass Index (BMI)	Decrease
Increase Body Surface Area (BSA)	Decrease
Adding flush	Increase
Increase contrast injection rate	Increase
Increase contrast iodine concentration	Increase
Alter contrast osmolality	No change

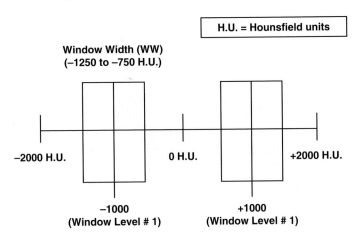

Window Level (WL) is the center line of Window Width (WW)

FIGURE 2.8. Illustration of the concept of windowing. The computed tomographic (CT) image represents the combination of the CT numbers and the chosen window settings (Reproduced with permission from Pelberg R, Mazur W. *Cardiac CT Angiography Manual*. London: Springer; 2007).

2.8 Windowing

Since the human eye cannot distinguish among more than about 500 shades of gray, windowing is necessary to reduce the number of shades of gray depicted on the computer screen. The window width (WW) is the range of gray-scale values displayed on the screen. The total CT number range or HU scale is from –2,000 to +2,000. The window level (WL) is the center of the selected WW. Alterations in the WL place emphasis on specific tissue types since all CT numbers lower than the lower limit of the WW will be displayed as black and all CT numbers higher than the upper limit of the WW will be displayed as white (Fig. 2.8).

2.9 Image Axes

Traditional axes are assigned to the CT image to help orient the reader. The X- and Y-axes' are the in-plane (axial) axes

IMAGE AXES

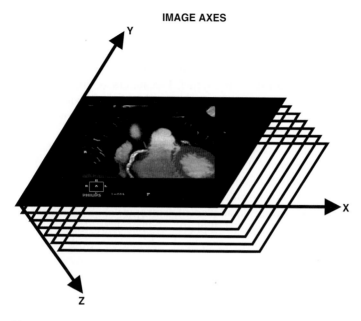

FIGURE 2.9. Cartoon to help visualize the various axes of a computed tomographic (CT) image. The X- and Y-axes' are the in-plane axes while the Z-axis is the through-plane axis (Reproduced from Pelberg R, Mazur W. *Cardiac CT Angiography Manual.* London: Springer; 2007).

and the Z-axis is the through-plane (head to toe or longitudinal) axis (Fig. 2.9).

2.10 Temporal Resolution

The temporal resolution is directly related to the gantry rotation speed. The most modern scanners have a gantry rotation time of ≤330 ms. Since a half gantry rotation is all that is required to completely image the heart, the effective temporal resolution of most scanners is ≤160 ms. With special reconstruction algorithms such as multisegment reconstruction, the temporal resolution may be reduced to ≤80 ms. Temporal resolution is most pertinent in cardiac CT angiography since most other vascular CT applications image vessels that are not rapidly moving (ascending aorta is a notable exception).

2.11 Spatial Resolution

The in-plane (X- and Y-axes') spatial resolution is determined by the specific characteristics of each CT scanner. The current spatial resolution of modern CT scanners is approximately 0.4 mm. The through-plane spatial resolution (Z-axis) is determined by both the detector width and the collimator width and is presently in the range of 0.6 mm.

The Z-axis resolution is important since it permits the creation of thinner CT slices. Despite increasing the noise and the radiation dose, thinner CT slices improve the Z-axis spatial resolution and allow the creation of isotropic voxels (voxels of similar dimensions in all planes). Isotropic voxels allow manipulation of the image in all planes without distortion.

Narrowing the detector and collimation width will also improve the X- and Y-axes' spatial resolution. However, detector size has currently been maximized and narrower collimation will force an unacceptable rise in the radiation dose necessary to penetrate the collimator. Thus, effective doses would be too high. Therefore, at the present time, spatial resolution has been optimized.

2.12 Collimation

Two types of collimation exist. Pre-patient collimators reside after the x-ray source but before the patient. They are used to shape the x-ray beam and to help avoid unnecessary x-ray exposure to the patient. Detector collimators reside immediately before the detector and help to prevent scattered x-ray photons from reaching the detector. In addition to thin CT slices, narrow collimation is also necessary to permit the creation of isotropic voxels.

2.13 Filtering

Image filters (also called kernels) are needed because the HU density of a particular pixel is not a discreet value but rather a Gaussian curve estimate. To improve the estimation of a particular voxel's HU density estimation, data are shared from neighboring voxels. The degree to which data from neighboring voxels are used determines the filter type. A sharp filter uses little data from neighboring voxels and thus the image is sharp and noisy. These filters are used to enhance anatomic edges. Smooth filters utilize more information from neighboring voxels and are used to reduce image noise. These filters result in smoother edges. Medium filters result in smoother are most common for routine use (Fig. 2.10). The name of each specific filter is company specific.

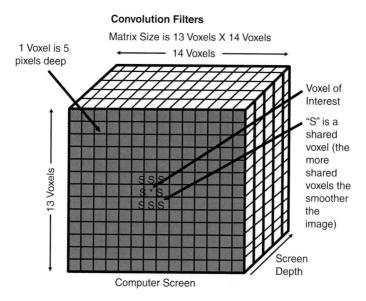

FIGURE 2.10. Demonstration of the concept of filtering. Filtering is necessary since computed tomographic (CT) densities are Gaussian curves and not exact numbers. To enhance the confidence of a particular density within one single voxel, sharing information from surrounding voxels is required. The degree to which this surrounding voxel information is used determines the filter type. Filters are also called kernels (Reproduced from Pelberg R, Mazur W. *Cardiac CT Angiography Manual*. London: Springer; 2007).

2.14 Pitch

Pitch is the term used for the movement of the patient table through the gantry. Pitch = table feed per rotation (mm)/coverage (mm). A pitch of 1 creates no gaps and no overlap in the data slabs. A pitch of less than 1 leads to overlapping image slabs, which is necessary for cardiac CT angiography but leads to the greater radiation exposure seen in cardiac CT imaging versus body CT imaging. A pitch of greater than 1 leads to gaps in the data set (Figs. 2.11 and 2.12).

2.15 Triggering

Cardiac CT angiography requires electrocardiographic triggering or gating. Peripheral vascular CT angiography only requires triggering if the ascending aorta is of particular interest since the ascending aorta is the only peripheral vascular artery that demonstrates significant motion. Two triggering types may be utilized. Prospective triggering is when the x-ray tube is powered on only during preselected cardiac phases and is turned off in between these phases. This reduces radiation greatly but eliminates the

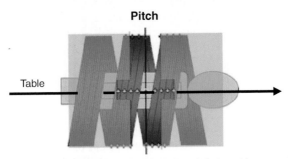

Pitch is term used for the speed with which the table moves through the gantry.

$$Pitch = \frac{Table\ Feed\ per\ rotation\ (mm)}{Coverage\ (mm)}$$

FIGURE 2.11. Cartoon illustrating the concept of pitch.

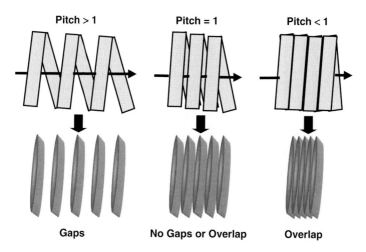

FIGURE 2.12. Effect of varying the pitch.

possibility for dynamic analyses. This type of gating is used for calcium scoring and for axial scanning (Fig. 2.13).

Retrospective triggering is used for spiral scanning techniques. Here, the x-ray tube is on during the entire scan time resulting in continuous scanning. Phases are then chosen for reconstruction after the scan takes place (retrospectively). This type of triggering results in a greater radiation dose but allows dynamic analyses since data exist during all physiologic time points (Fig. 2.14).

2.16 Post-Processing Techniques

Multiple post-processing techniques are available to the reader to aid in image analysis. The Volume Rendered Technique (VRT) or Three-Dimensional VRT (3D VRT) (Fig. 2.15) uses shading and color coding to present anatomical structures in a 3D display. This reconstruction should only be used for general anatomical analysis. It is helpful among other things to efficiently evaluate the vasculature, to locate

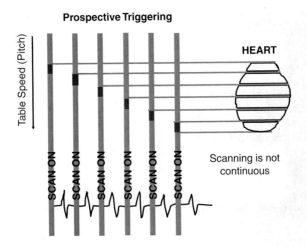

FIGURE 2.13. Demonstration of the concept of prospective triggering (Reproduced with permission from Pelberg R, Mazur W. *Cardiac CT Angiography Manual*. London: Springer; 2007).

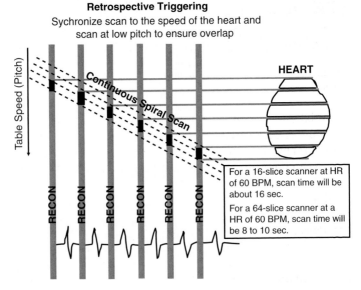

FIGURE 2.14. Illustration of the concept of retrospective triggering (Reproduced with permission from Pelberg R, Mazur W. *Cardiac CT Angiography Manual*. London: Springer; 2007).

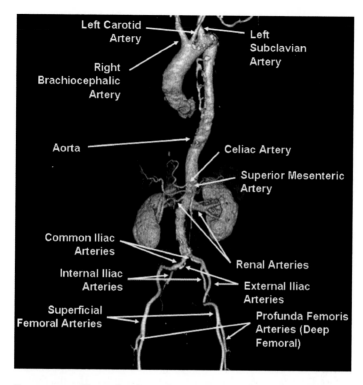

FIGURE 2.15. Example of a volume-rendered (VRT, 3D) image of the aorta and its major branches.

potential points of interest, to identify aneurysms, to gain an overview of endovascular stents and to follow the course of peripheral bypass grafts. This technique should never be used to make or confirm a diagnosis since the image may be markedly altered by the window settings.

Multiplanar reformatting (MPR) is a technique where image planes of one slice thick are analyzed. The Hounsfield unit density of the voxels in this chosen plane is viewed on the screen. Oblique MPR is most sensitive for finding and characterizing lesions. However, small vessels and structures are very difficult to track in multiple planes using this reformatting technique since only very short segments of vasculature are visible on the screen at once. MPR is used to hone in on a suspected problem for further analysis and for confirmation (Fig. 2.16).

Depiction of Oblique MPR

In this cartoon, each voxel is composed of 10 slices deep into the screen (in a 512 X 512 matrix there would be 512 voxels across the screen and 512 voxels down the screen).

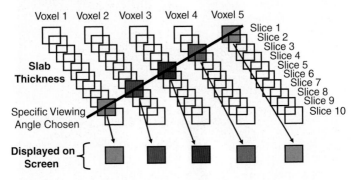

FIGURE 2.16. Illustration in cartoon format of the concept of multi-planar reformatting (MPR) (Reproduced with permission from Pelberg R, Mazur W. *Cardiac CT Angiography Manual*. London: Springer; 2007).

Maximum intensity projections (MIP) are multiple slices thick. Structures may be viewed in any chosen plane. The thickness of the reconstruction is also selected by the reader. The maximum intensity or brightest pixel anywhere within the chosen thickness is projected forward and displayed on the screen. The exact location of this intensity within the thickness is unknown. MIP is the most practical method of navigating through small structures and arteries because longer segments are visualized on the screen at once. However, as the MIP thickness increases, the sensitivity for detecting a lesion is reduced. Thin MIP is a technique where the chosen thickness is very close to the thickness of the structure of interest and is the most practical method of over-reading and navigating the data set while maintaining adequate sensitivity to find areas that require further analysis (Figs. 2.17 and 2.18).

Curved MPR (cMPR) projects a single line of densities in any plane or planes chosen by the reader across the data set and displays them on the screen in one plane. This technique may be useful as long as the reader recognizes the potential downfalls which include poorly visualized branch vessels and the possibility of introducing artifacts into the image (Fig. 2.19).

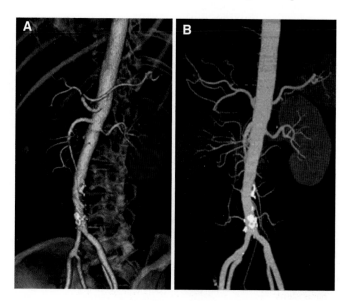

FIGURE 2.17. Panel A is another example of a volume-rendered (VRT) image of the descending aorta and its major branches. Panel B is a maximum intensity projection (MIP) of the same anatomy.

Depiction of MIP

In this cartoon, each voxel depicted on the computer screen is 5 slices thick. If the screen is a 512 X 512 matrix, there would be 512 voxels across the screen and 512 voxels down the screen. MIP format identifies the brightest point in the slab thickness within each voxel and projects this density forward to be viewed on the screen.

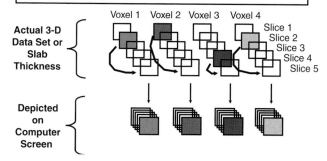

FIGURE 2.18. Diagram explaining maximum intensity projections (MIPs) (Reproduced with permission from Pelberg R, Mazur W. *Cardiac CT Angiography Manual*. London: Springer; 2007).

24   Chapter 2.   CT Basics

Depiction of Curved MPR

In this cartoon, each voxel depicted on the computer screen is 10 slices thick. If the screen is a 512 by 512 matrix, there would be 512 voxels across the screen and 512 voxels down the screen. The curved MPR format projects a single, user defined, line through the image in any number of chosen planes and displays this curved line onto the computer screen as a single plane of voxel densities. Since this is an MPR format, the resulting image is one plane thick.

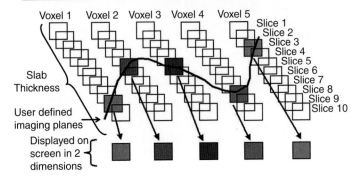

FIGURE 2.19. Illustration of the concept of a curved multiplanar reformatting (cMPR) (Reproduced with permission from Pelberg R, Mazur W. *Cardiac CT Angiography Manual*. London: Springer; 2007).

Chapter 3
Concepts in Radiation

Many of the concepts and sections in this chapter were excerpted from the first book in this series, *Cardiac CT Angiography Manual*.[1] This chapter is rewritten to be more inclusive and up to date.

3.1 Definitions

Radiation: Defined as energy in transit.
Ionizing radiation: Defined as high energy in transit that can remove electrons from an atom.
Radioactivity: The characteristic of a material to emit ionizing radiation.

3.2 Types of Radiation

Various types of radiation are listed in Table 3.1.

3.3 Electromagnetic Spectrum

X-rays and gamma rays are part of the electromagnetic spectrum (Fig. 3.1) unlike alpha and beta radiation which are radiation particles and not electromagnetic waves. Other members of the electromagnetic spectrum in order of

R. Pelberg, W. Mazur, *Vascular CT Angiography Manual*,
DOI: 10.1007/978-1-84996-260-5_3,
© Springer-Verlag London Limited 2011

TABLE 3.1. Various types of radiation and their characteristics.

Types of radiation			
Radiation type	Description	Charge	Shielding material
Alpha	Particle	+2	Skin, clothes
Beta	Particle	+1	Plastic, glass
Gamma	Electromagnetic wave	0	Lead, concrete
X-ray	Electromagnetic wave	0	Lead, concrete

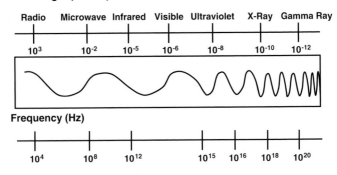

FIGURE 3.1. Electromagnetic spectrum. The higher the frequency, the higher the energy of the electromagnetic wave.

decreasing frequency include ultraviolet light, visible light, infrared, microwaves and radio waves.

Gamma rays are produced by unstable nuclei while x-rays emanate from the atom's electron shell. Gamma rays have a higher frequency than x-rays and thus have slightly more energy. Alpha and beta particles have significantly more energy than x-rays or gamma rays but have very weak penetration ability (shielded by skin or clothing). On the contrary, x-rays and gamma rays have a remarkable ability to penetrate (shielded only by lead or concrete).

3.4 X-Ray Production

Medical x-rays are produced in an x-ray tube (Fig. 3.2) which consists of a negative cathode and a positive, rotating anode. The cathode and anode are made of tungsten. The cathode is heated which repels its composition electrons. Positive charge is then applied to the anode to create a current which separates the electrons from the cathode and accelerates them toward the anode. The velocity with which these electrons travel toward the anode depends on the charge difference applied to the anode.

These cathode-generated electrons strike the anode, interact with its inner electron shells and consequently produce characteristic x-ray photons. Characteristic x-ray photons occur when an incident electron strikes the inner shells of the anode with enough energy to displace an electron. Consequently, a separate outer shell electron then moves inward to replace the vacant inner shell. The remaining energy from this interaction is emitted as a characteristic x-ray photon (Fig. 3.3).

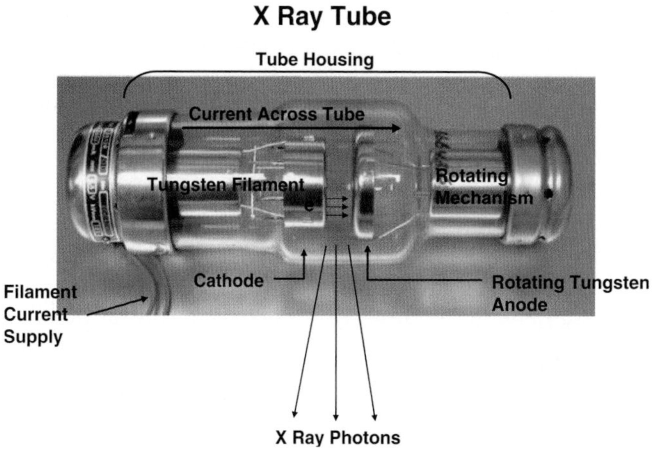

X Ray Tube

FIGURE 3.2. Basic x-ray tube.

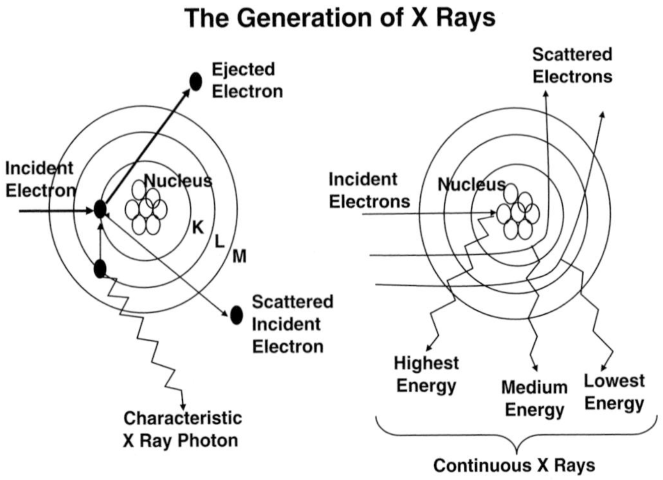

The Generation of X Rays

FIGURE 3.3. Production of characteristic x-ray photons (important for computed tomographic [CT] imaging) and continuous x-rays (enemy of CT imaging). Characteristic x-ray photons are produced when the incident photon interacts with an inner shell electron, causing it to be ejected from the atom. An electron from an outer shell then moves downward to fill the vacant inner shell and the resulting energy difference is emitted as a characteristic x-ray photon. The initial electron is scattered. Continuous x-rays are produced when incident x-rays are merely scattered but do not cause the ejection of the inner shell electron. The shell with which the incident photon interacts determines the energy of the continuous x-rays.

The charge difference applied between the anode and the cathode determines the energy (measured in kilo electron volts, keV) of the characteristic x-ray photons produced by the x-ray tube. The photon flux (measured in milliamperes, mA) describes the number of x-rays produced by the x-ray tube per unit time and is a function of applied current.

Unlike characteristic x-rays, continuous x-rays (Fig. 3.3) are not applicable to medicine. These occur when the incident electron does not displace an electron but merely interacts with it. The energy change that results is emitted as a continuous x-ray, the energy of which depends on the type of electron to electron interaction that occurs, which in turn is based on the speed with which the incident electrons strike the anode.

3.5 Quantifying Radiation

Activity is defined as the number of times per second a radioactive material decays and releases radiation.

Radiation may be quantified in terms meaningful to the human body and in terms related to the computed tomography (CT) machine settings themselves. Terms designed to quantify radiation as it relates to its effects on the human body include exposure, absorbed dose, equivalent dose and effective dose.

Exposure is the measure of the ionization produced in air by x-rays or gamma rays.

Absorbed dose is the amount of radiation energy absorbed into a given mass of tissue.

Equivalent dose is the energy per unit mass multiplied by an adjustment factor for the type or quality of radiation. X-rays and gamma rays have a radiation adjustment factor of 1 so that for x-rays and gamma rays, absorbed dose equals equivalent dose. Alpha particles, on the other hand, have an adjustment factor of 20.

Effective dose is the sum of all weighted equivalent doses in all the exposed organs and tissues of the body and is measured in Sieverts (Sv). Effective dose compares the cancer risk of a non-uniform exposure of ionizing radiation with the risks caused by a uniform exposure to the whole body. Effective dose = equivalent dose × tissue weighting factor. The tissue weighting factor is tissue-specific and is represented as a fraction such that the effective dose is a portion of the equivalent dose and is therefore only a dose estimate. It may be an underestimation.

Effective dose may also be calculated from the equation, effective dose = DLP × k. DLP is the dose-length product and is derived by the equation, DLP = CTDIw × scan length and has units mSv·cm. The constant k is related to the area of the body being scanned. For the chest, k = 0.017. The units of k are mSv/mSv·cm so that the units of effective dose are in mSv. Table 3.2 lists the k values for various body regions.

The units of these various body-specific radiation terms are listed in Table 3.3.

Radiation dose may also be quantified in terms of scanner-specific characteristics and settings. To quantify the CT scanner–specific radiation dose (not the patient dose), the following terms are used; computed tomography dose index (CTDI), weighted (CTDIw) and CTDIvol.

Computed tomography dose index (*CTDI*): Estimate of the delivered dose for the given specific scan parameters (keV, mAs, etc.). It is measured in a thermolucent dosimeter (Fig. 3.4).

TABLE 3.2. k Values for various body regions.

k is a constant reflecting the radiation sensitivity of a particular body part.

Body part	k
Head	0.0023
Neck	0.0056
Chest	0.017
Abdomen	0.015
Pelvis	0.019

TABLE 3.3. Various radiation units characterizing multiple radiation terms.

	Radiation units		
	Old unit	SI unit	Conversions
Exposure	Roentgen (R)	Coulomb/kg (C/kg)	1 R = 258 (µC/kg)
Absorbed	Rad (rad)	Gray (Gy)	1 Gy = 100 rad
Equivalentdose	Rem (rem)	Sievert (Sv)	1 Sv = 100 rem
Activity	Curie (Ci)	Becquerel (Bq)	1 mCi = 37 mBq

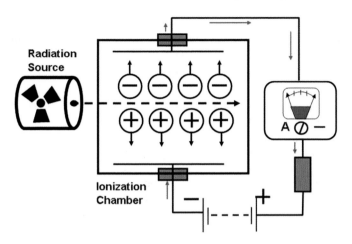

FIGURE 3.4. Thermolucent ionization chamber used for calculating the computed tomography dose index (CTDI).

Weighted CTDI (CTDIw): The weighted average of the CTDI in the X- and Y-planes. CTDIw = 2/3 CTDI surface + 1/3 CTDI center. The units for CTDI and CTDIw are Gray (Gy). In the case of x-rays, Gy are equivalent to Sv since the conversion factor is 1.

CTDI and CTDIw do not account for scan length (Z-axis).

CTDIvol: Constructed to account for the Z-axis (scan length). CTDIvol = CTDIw/pitch. As the pitch decreases, the scan length increases; so the CTDIvol will increase. The unit of CTDIvol is also Gy. DLP is also a scanner-specific dose estimation term. It is the best scanner-specific dose estimate available.

3.6 Understanding Milliamperes

The term mA (milliamperes) does not take into account scan time. Thus, the term mAs (milliamperes-seconds) was created to account for scan time. For a pitch of 1, mAs = mA × gantry rotation time. In cardiac CT, a pitch of less than 1 is required for the necessary image overlap. Therefore, for a pitch of less than 1, the term mAs$_{eff}$ (effective mAs) is used. Effective mAs is calculated using the equation mAs$_{eff}$ = mAs × exposure time, where exposure time = gantry rotation time/pitch. Therefore, mAs$_{eff}$ = mAs × gantry rotation time/pitch.

3.7 Radiation Exposure

In the USA, the background radiation dose is 3 mSv per year. Radon accounts for 52% of all low-energy transmissions (LETS, where LETS = <100 mSv). Cosmic sources represent 12% of all LETS. Background radiation is responsible for 82% of all patient radiation. Air travel exposes a person to 0.01 mSv per 1,000 miles traveled and cigarette smoking exposes the smoker to 2.8 mSv per year. The effective dose of a mammogram is 0.13 mSv. Doses from other common medical examinations are found in Fig. 3.5.

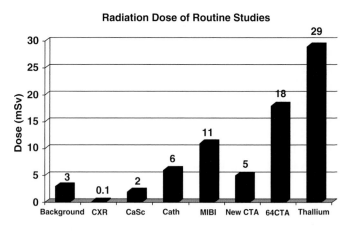

FIGURE 3.5. Illustration in graph form of the radiation doses for various commonly ordered imaging studies as well as background radiation levels. New CTA refers to newer cardiac computed tomographic (CT) angiography techniques using prospective imaging and other radiation sparing protocols.

Man-made, medical radiation accounts for 18% of all human radiation exposure. Of the 18% medical, human radiation exposure, 58% is from an x-ray source and 21% is from nuclear medicine.

Radiation may cause damage to DNA. These effects are either direct or indirect via free radical generation. Radiation effects on the body are classified as *deterministic* (acute) or *stochastic* (chronic) effects. Deterministic effects are threshold and dose-dependent and include rash, nausea and emesis. *Stochastic* effects are based on the cumulative radiation dose over time and include cancer and cataracts.

The most widely accepted theory regarding the risk of radiation is the *linear, no threshold dose–response theory* (Fig. 3.6) which states that there is no threshold radiation dose for potential radiation damage and the risk for radiation-induced side effects increases linearly with rising dose. Rapidly dividing cells are most susceptible to radiation

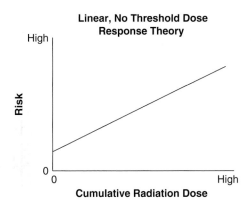

FIGURE 3.6. Graph depicting the linear, no threshold dose–response theory regarding radiation exposure. This theory is the most widely regarded and states that the risk of radiation exposure increases linearly with dose and there is no threshold where this risk begins. A risk exists at a dose of zero because all persons are exposed to background radiation which also carries some risk.

damage and thus an unborn child is at great risk. The maximum allowable radiation exposure during pregnancy is 5 mSv over 9 months. This translates to 500 mRem over 9 months, not to exceed 50 mRem per month.

Radiation dose should always be kept to a minimum. Always think *ALARA* (as low as reasonably achievable). Methods to reduce radiation dose include reducing keV. This is extremely effective (70% reduction) because radiation dose is proportional to the square of the keV. Using axial scanning (prospective triggering) will reduce the radiation dose by nearly 80%. Electrocardiogram (ECG) dose modulation will reduce the dose by nearly 50%. Dose modulation is used mainly in cardiac CT. Other parameters that may be adjusted to reduce radiation dose are noted in Fig. 3.7.

Factors Influencing Radiation Dose

- **Voltage Setting (KV):** increasing the voltage increases the dose thus increasing the risk
  - dose increases proportional to the square of the KV so this is the most effective way to reduce dose of all options listed here.
- **Current (mA):** increasing the mA increases the dose proportionally so the risk increases. Adjusted manually or automatically with ECG Tube Current Modulation.
- **Slice Thickness:** decreasing the slice thickness increases the dose (more radiation per slice) and therefore increases the risk.
- **Pitch:** reducing the pitch increases the dose (increased scan time) therefore increases the risk.
- **Scan Time:** anything that increases scan time increases the dose and the risk.
- **Selected Field of View:** increasing the selected FOV increases dose and risk.
- **Beam Focus:** the less beam focus the greater the unnecessary radiation exposure and the greater the risk.
- **Scatter:** the more scatter the more risk.

FIGURE 3.7. List of factors that influence radiation dose and thus risk to the patient.

Chapter 4
Technical Aspects of Vascular CT Angiography

Vascular computed tomographic (CT) angiography is a less complicated technique than cardiac CT angiography since for the most part the structures of interest are static. The key to vascular CT angiography is to optimize contrast opacification at the point of interest at the time that the region of interest is scanned. To succeed, protocols must allow optimal contrast timing. This requires coordinating the appropriate volume of contrast over the appropriate time at the appropriate rate of injection. While with cardiac CT angiography both the test bolus and bolus tracking techniques are both employed to appropriately time the scan after contrast injection, vascular CT angiography most often employs bolus tracking where a strategic region of interest is selected depending on the scan type and imaging begins when the Hounsfield units (HU) within the selected region of interest reach a predetermined threshold.

The injection system most often utilized for peripheral CT angiography is a dual lumen injection system where contrast injection is followed by a saline chaser bolus to wash out the contrast and tighten the contrast bolus. This technique also reduces the contrast load and improves the iodine flux (increasing the contrast effect).

While gating to the electrocardiogram is most often not necessary, retrospective scanning with electrocardiographic gating is suggested when imaging the thoracic aorta to avoid motion artifact since this region of the aorta does move

R. Pelberg, W. Mazur, *Vascular CT Angiography Manual*,
DOI: 10.1007/978-1-84996-260-5_4,
© Springer-Verlag London Limited 2011

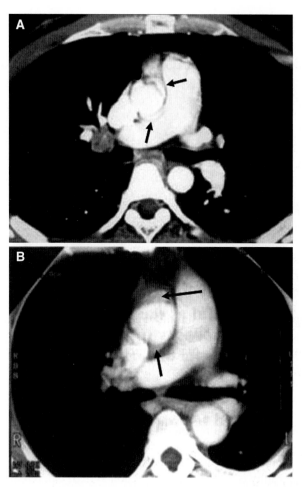

FIGURE 4.1. Panels A and B demonstrate two separate examples of motion artifact at the level of the ascending aorta, which may mimic an ascending aortic dissection (*black arrows*). Since the ascending aorta moves rapidly with each heart beat, gated, retrospective imaging is used when the ascending aorta is the focus to help eliminate this motion artifact. A clue that these findings are artifactual is the symmetrical nature of the suspected abnormality. When present, motion artifact in the ascending aorta appears on exact opposite sides of the aorta in the axial plane as shown above. Rarely does a dissection flap demonstrate this symmetrical appearance.

during the cardiac cycle and is thus prone to artifact (may mimic aortic dissection, Fig. 4.1). Disadvantages of retrospective gating include increased radiation, increased scan planning complexity, and decreased patient throughput. Prospective triggering without electrocardiogram gating suffices for most of other applications.

Slice thickness may vary depending on the scan indication. For example, the narrowest slice thickness should be used when evaluating for dissection to help identify the flap. Narrowing the slice thickness will serve to improve the spatial resolution in the Z plane, thus improving the ability to differentiate small structures such as dissection flaps.

Narrow slice thicknesses may not be necessary for evaluation of aortic aneurysms or for other indications not requiring such fine detail resolution.

Imaging protocols are relatively standard and straightforward. While many protocols may allow successful imaging, the following imaging protocols are listed below for reference. The protocols used in our laboratory to a large degree were shared with us by Dr. Peter Fail at the Cardiology Institute of the South, a recognized leader in the field of vascular imaging and intervention.

4.1 Protocols (Table 4.1)

For all scanning protocols the keV is set to 120–150 and the mAs are optimized to the scanner type and to the patient size. Larger patients may require higher mAs. A typical pitch of 1–1.5 is applied, resulting in small spaces (0.75–1 mm) between slices. Contrary to cardiac CT angiography where slice overlap is mandatory, peripheral CT angiography does not require overlapping image slices.

A pregnancy test is recommended before routine scans in woman of child-bearing age. Pregnancy testing is deferred in emergency cases where the risk-benefit ratio favors performing the scan emergently. Screening for renal function and iodine contrast allergies is also mandatory.

TABLE 4.1. This table depicts the CT protocols for common vascular CT angiogram studies.

Study type	Contrast volume	Injection rate	Bolus tracking ROI and threshold	Slice thickness	Scan field
Carotid, vertebral, subclavian, and axillary	75 ml	5 ml/s	Aortic arch 180 HU	0.75 mm	Below the aortic arch to top of the head
Thoracic aorta (not ascending aorta)	100 ml	3 ml/s	Aortic arch 180 HU	0.75 mm (dissection) and 1–2 mm (other)	Above the aortic arch to below the bifurcation of the internal and external iliac arteries
Ascending aorta (gated scan)	100 ml	3 ml/s	Aortic arch 180 HU	0.75 mm	Above the aortic arch through the adrenal glands
Aorto-femoral with run-off (CT angio of lower extremities)	125 ml	3 ml/s	Descending thoracic aorta 180 HU	≤1 mm	Above diaphragm to the feet
Thoracic and abdominal aorta with run-off	125 ml	3 ml/s	Aortic arch 180 HU	≤1 mm	Apex of the chest to the feet
CT upper extremity arterial	100 ml	4 ml/s	Aortic arch 180 HU	≤1 mm	Aortic arch including the arm

CT for pulmonary embolism	75 ml	5 ml/s	Pulmonary artery 80 HU	0.75 mm	Apex of chest to below the diaphragm
Abdominal aorta	100 ml	3 ml/s	Descending thoracic aorta 180 HU	0.5 mm (if MMS is used)	Above the diaphragm to below the bifurcation of the internal and external iliac arteries
Renal artery	100ml(CRI−) 40ml(CRI+)	3 ml/s	Descending thoracic aorta 180 HU	≤1 mm	Above renals to iliacs (CRI−). Include only renals(CRI+)

4.1.1 Carotid, Vertebral, Subclavian, and Axillary Arteries

Common indications for carotid CT angiography include bruit, syncope, dizziness, vertigo, abnormal ultrasound evaluation, planning for carotid endarterectomy (CEA), diplopia, visual disturbance, amaurosis fugax, and ataxia. Arm claudication and embolic phenomenon to the hand are the indications often used for subclavian and axillary artery scanning. Unfortunately, since flow velocity and direction cannot be directly measured by CT angiography, the subclavian steal syndrome cannot be reliably identified with CT.

The field of view (FOV) includes just below the aortic arch to the top of the head. Isovue 370 contrast is injected at 5 ml/s. Bolus tracking is utilized with a region of interest in the aortic arch. The scan begins when the contrast in the aortic arch reaches 180 HU. Apply the thinnest possible collimation (0.75 mm).

4.1.2 Thoracic Aorta Excluding the Ascending Aorta

Common indications include thoracic aortic aneurysm, abdominal aortic aneurysm, aortic dissection, atypical chest pain, coarctation of the aorta, other congenital diseases of the aorta, persistent left superior vena cava, interrupted inferior vena cava, and suspected pulmonary embolism. An advantage of CT angiography over invasive angiography for these indications is that intramural hematoma can be identified with CT technology.

The FOV for this imaging protocol extends from above the aortic arch and ends below the bifurcation of the internal and external iliac arteries. Inject 100 ml of Isovue 370 at 3 ml/s using bolus tracking with a region of interest placed at the level of the aortic arch. The scan begins when the contrast in the aortic arch reaches 180 HU. Often a slice thickness of 1–2 mm may be used to reduce radiation. If dissection is suspected, slice thicknesses of 0.75 mm may be more appropriate to improve Z-plane spatial resolution.

4.1.3 Ascending Aorta

Common indications include ascending aortic aneurysm, aortic dissection, and congenital disease of the aorta.

The FOV begins above the aortic arch and ends through the adrenal glands. Beta-blockers are used to lower the heart rate, if possible, since electrocardiographic (ECG) gating is necessary. For this reason, retrospective, helical imaging is utilized. Inject 100 ml of Isovue 370 at 3 ml/s. Bolus tracking with a region of interest at the level of the aortic arch is used. The contrast threshold is set at 180 HU. This protocol is performed in a similar fashion as cardiac CT angiography since retrospective, gated imaging is used to eliminate motion of the ascending aorta. Slice thicknesses of 1–2 mm are used. Again, if dissection is suspected, thinner slice thicknesses, such as 0.75 mm, are recommended.

Delayed scans may be used (2 min after injection) to allow visualization of a late filling false lumen, slow endoleaks, or contrast extravasation from a rupture.

4.1.4 Aorta with Ilio-Femoral Run-Off (CT Angiography Lower Extremities)

Common indications include abdominal aortic aneurysm, claudication and peripheral vascular disease, abnormal ankle-brachial index (ABI), lower extremity pain, lower extremity numbness and weakness, stent patency, peripheral arterial aneurysm such as in the iliac, femoral, and popliteal arteries, and preoperative assessment and postoperative surveillance of lower extremity bypass grafts.

The FOV begins above the diaphragm and extends through the feet. Inject 125 ml of Isovue 370 at 3 ml/s. Use bolus tracking with a region of interest in the descending thoracic aorta above the diaphragm with a threshold of 180 HU. Slice thicknesses of less than or equal to 1 mm are used.

It is always wise to preset a salvage scan (delayed scan) protocol to be employed if the initial scan inadvertently outruns the contrast (no contrast seen below the knees). By activating the delayed scan protocol, a repeat imaging sequence is performed from the knees through the feet at the push of a button. This safeguard may potentially salvage a spoiled scan.

4.1.5 Thoracic and Abdominal Aorta with Ilio-Femoral Run-Off (Evaluation of Axillary-Bifemoral Bypass Grafts)

Common indications include the evaluation of axillary-bifemoral bypass grafts. Other indications overlap with those listed in the aorta with ilio-femoral run-off protocol (CT angiography lower extremities).

The FOV begins at the apex of the chest above graft insertions and ends through the feet. Inject 125 ml of Isovue 370 at 3 ml/s. Bolus tracking is used with a region of interest in the aortic arch using a threshold of 180 HU. Use a slice thickness of less than or equal to 1 mm.

4.1.6 CT Venography of the Upper Extremity

Common indications include any reason to demonstrate patency of the axillary, subclavian, and ulnar veins.

Inject 100 ml of Isovue 370 at 2 ml/s. Place the intravenous access in the hand of the affected side. For bilateral venous opacification, inject both hands simultaneously using a Y extension catheter. Here the scan may begin almost immediately. The usual slice thickness is 1 mm.

4.1.7 CT Angiography of the Upper extremity (Not Venography and Not Thoracic Outlet)

Common indications include embolus, thrombosis, dialysis graft assessment, central line, swelling, pain, and tenderness.

Inject 100 ml of Isovue 370 at 4 ml/s. Use bolus tracking with a region of interest placed in the aortic arch. Trigger the scan when the contrast in the region of interest reaches 180 HU. Place the intravenous access in the opposite extremity of the affected limb to avoid venous contamination. This study is technically difficult to perform bilaterally. Use a slice thickness of less than or equal to 1 mm.

4.1.8 CT Venography for Lower Extremity Vein Mapping (Not for DVT)

This scan requires a foot injection of 125 ml of Isovue 370 at 2 ml/s using a power injector. Begin the scan without significant delay. The slice thickness is usually 1 mm.

4.1.9 CT Chest for Pulmonary Embolus

Inject 75 ml of Isovue 370 at 4 ml/s using a slice thickness of 0.75 mm or less. Bolus tracking is used with a region of interest in the pulmonary artery. Begin the scan when the contrast in the region of interest reaches 180 HU. Be sure the FOV includes the lung apices and extends below the diaphragm.

4.1.10 CT Chest for Thoracic Outlet Syndrome

This protocol is used specifically when thoracic outlet syndrome is suspected.

Inject 100 ml of Isovue 370 at 5 ml/s. Scan the patient with the arms down and then re-scan with the arms above the head to dynamically evaluate the subclavian arterial flow. Use a slice thickness of 1 mm.

4.1.11 CT of the Abdominal Aorta

Common indications include abdominal aortic aneurysm, aortic dissection, renal artery stenosis, potential kidney donor, mesenteric ischemia, renal or splenic artery aneurysm, visceral artery aneurysm, and pre- and post-evaluation of a liver transplant patient.

Inject 100 ml of Isovue 370 at 3 ml/s. Use bolus tracking to time the scan with the region of interest in the descending thoracic aorta. Begin the scan when the contrast in the region of interest reaches 180 HU. If using the Medical Metrx Solutions (MMS) for endovascular stent graft planning, use a narrow slice thickness of 0.5 mm. The FOV ranges from above the diaphragm to below the internal–external iliac bifurcations.

When performing the imaging exam to assess an aortic stent graft, perform a pre-contrast scan prior to the study and a repeat scan 5 min after the contrasted scan to exclude slow endoleaks.

4.1.12 Renal Artery Stenosis Protocol

This protocol is performed to evaluate for renal artery stenosis.

If contrast-related complications are not a worry, inject 100 ml of Isovue 370 at 3 ml/s. The FOV will include the entire aorta from above the upper poles of both kidneys including the celiac and superior mesenteric arteries through the bifurcation of the internal and external iliac arteries. Bolus tracking is used to time the scan, placing the region of interest in the descending thoracic aorta. Begin the scan when the contrast in the region of interest reaches 180 HU. Use a slice thickness of 1 mm or less. If contrast-induced nephropathy is an issue, scan only from upper poles of kidneys to the bottom of the kidneys using only 40 ml contrast.

4.2 Issues Regarding Renal Insufficiency

We recommend that the physician be notified prior to scheduling any CT angiogram if the creatinine is greater than 1.7 mg/dl, if the creatinine is greater than 1.5 mg/dl in a diabetic patient or if the blood urea nitrogen (BUN) is greater than 30 in a patient with diabetes. We require a BUN and creatinine be performed within 2 weeks of the imaging exam.

Metformin is always held for 48 h after the scan. In renal insufficiency, we discontinue the Metformin 24 h before the scan and hydrate the patient with 0.9% NS at 1 ml/kg for 6 h prior to the scan. We recommend prescribing mucomyst at a dose of 600 mg PO BID 1 day prior to the scan and continue for 1 day after the scan. Obtain a BUN and creatinine 1 day after the scan. In dialysis patients, the scan may be coordinated with dialysis.

4.3 Issues Regarding Iodinated Dye Allergies

We require a physician be notified prior to the scan if a contrast dye allergy is present. Many iodine contrast allergy protocols exist. We typically give 60 mg of prednisone the night before the scan and 60 mg of prednisone the morning of the scan. Administer 50 mg of benadryl intravenously 30 min prior to exam. If the scan is an emergency, 100 mg of intravenous hydrocortisone may be administered concomitantly with 50 mg of intravenous benadryl just before the test.

Chapter 5
Carotid and Upper Extremity CT Angiography

5.1 Anatomy (Figs. 5.1–5.3)

When beginning proximally, the normal aortic arch gives rise to the right brachiocephalic artery, the left carotid artery, and, finally, the left subclavian artery. The brachiocephalic artery

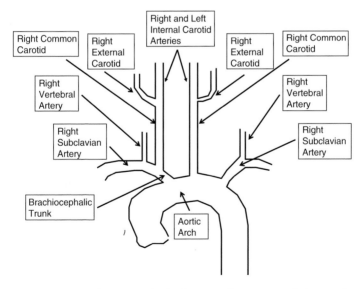

FIGURE 5.1. Depiction of the basic normal anatomy of the aortic arch and its great branch vessels. See text for description.

R. Pelberg, W. Mazur, *Vascular CT Angiography Manual*,
DOI: 10.1007/978-1-84996-260-5_5,
© Springer-Verlag London Limited 2011

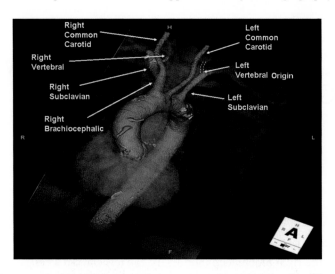

Figure 5.2. A volume-rendered, segmented, semitransparent illustration of a normal aortic arch and its great vessels and branches.

Figure 5.3. Panel A represents an axial image of the carotid and vertebral anatomy in the neck. RV: Right vertebral. RJV: Right jugular vein. RC: Right carotid artery. LC: Left carotid artery. LJV: Left jugular vein. LV: Left vertebral artery. Panel B illustrates an axial view superior to the bifurcation of the internal and external carotid arteries. Here the vertebral arteries are visualized as they course through the vertebral foramen. RIC: Right internal carotid artery. REC: Right external carotid artery. LEC: Left external carotid artery. LIC: Left internal carotid artery. *Single asterisk*: Right vertebral artery coursing through its foramen. *Double asterisk*: Left vertebral artery coursing through its foramen. The yellow "A", "P", "L" and "R" represent anterior, posterior, left and right respectively.

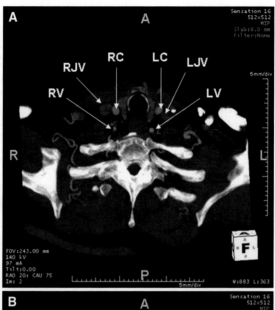

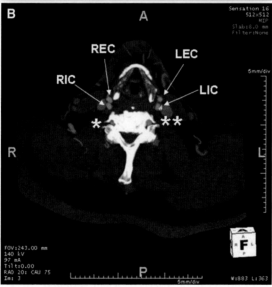

and the left carotid artery are more anterior on the arch. The right common carotid artery and right vertebral arteries arise from the right brachiocephalic artery. The right common carotid artery splits into the right internal and the right external carotid arteries. The left common carotid artery, arising directly from the aortic arch, gives rise to the left internal and the left external carotid artery. The carotid bulb (Fig. 5.4) refers to the region just before the bifurcation of the internal carotid artery. More distally on the arch, the left subclavian

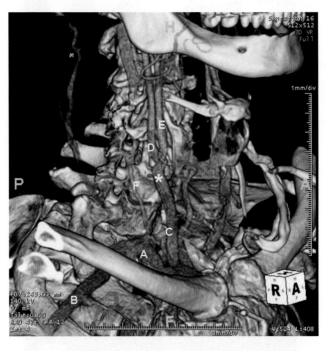

FIGURE 5.4. Demonstration of the location of the carotid bulb (*white asterisk*). A: Right brachiocephalic artery. B: Right subclavian artery. C: Right common carotid artery. D: Right internal carotid artery. E: Right external carotid artery. F: Right vertebral artery. The yellow "H," "F," "A," and "P" represent head, foot, anterior, and posterior respectively.

artery arises and gives off the left vertebral artery. Many normal variant arch anomalies can occur (Figs. 5.5–5.9).

The internal carotid arteries supply the anterior brain, the eye, the forehead, and the nose. It gives rise to many branches including the hypophyseal artery, ophthalmic artery, anterior cerebral artery, middle cerebral artery, and posterior communicating artery.

The external carotid artery arises anteriorly from the common carotid artery and gives rise to multiple facial branches including the anterior branches, posterior branches, ascending branches, and terminal branches. The anterior branches include the superior thyroid, lingual, and external maxillary arteries. The posterior branches are the occipital and posterior auricular arteries and the ascending branch includes the ascending pharyngeal artery. Finally, the terminal branches are the superficial temporal and internal maxillary arteries. The external

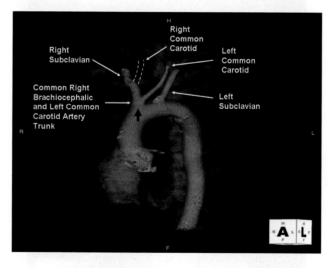

FIGURE 5.5. Illustration of a typical, normal variant, bovine aortic arch. With a bovine arch, the left carotid artery and the right brachiocephalic artery arise from a common trunk (*black arrow*).

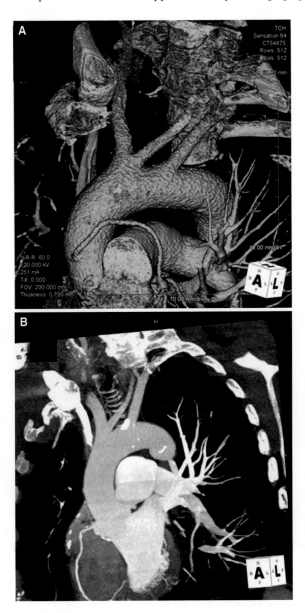

Figure 5.6. Another representation of a bovine aortic arch. Panel A is a volume-rendered image and panel B is a maximum intensity projection (MIP).

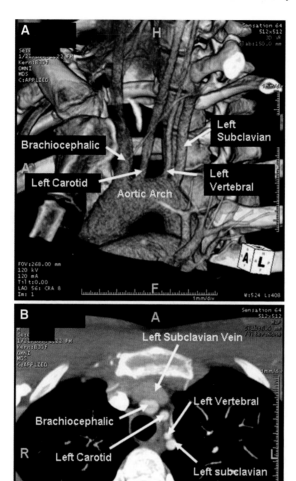

FIGURE 5.7. Depiction of a common anomaly where the left vertebral artery arises directly from the aortic arch instead of emanating
from the left subclavian artery. Panel A is a volume-rendered image
and panel B is an axial, maximum intensity projection (MIP).

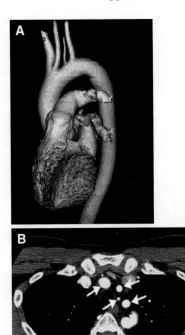

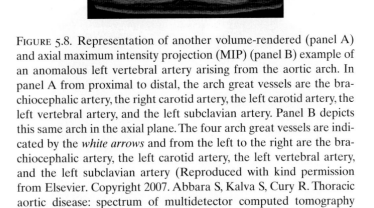

FIGURE 5.8. Representation of another volume-rendered (panel A) and axial maximum intensity projection (MIP) (panel B) example of an anomalous left vertebral artery arising from the aortic arch. In panel A from proximal to distal, the arch great vessels are the brachiocephalic artery, the right carotid artery, the left carotid artery, the left vertebral artery, and the left subclavian artery. Panel B depicts this same arch in the axial plane. The four arch great vessels are indicated by the *white arrows* and from the left to the right are the brachiocephalic artery, the left carotid artery, the left vertebral artery, and the left subclavian artery (Reproduced with kind permission from Elsevier. Copyright 2007. Abbara S, Kalva S, Cury R. Thoracic aortic disease: spectrum of multidetector computed tomography imaging findings. *J Cardiovasc Comput Tomogr.* 2007;1:40–54).

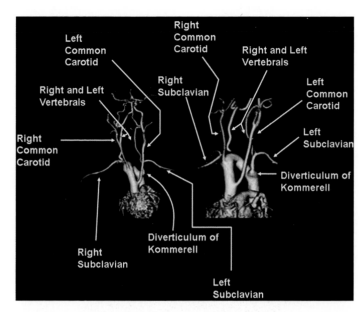

FIGURE 5.9. Illustration of a volume-rendered image of a cervical aortic arch which sits high in the thoracic cavity and may reside in the neck. In addition, a diverticulum of Kommerell is apparent. The embryological etiology of a cervical aortic arch is not entirely known (Reproduced with kind permission of Lippincott Williams & Wilkins. Copyright 2008. Poellinger A, Lembcke A, Elgeti T, et al. The cervical aortic arch: a rare vascular anomaly. *Circulation*. 2008;117:2716–2717).

carotid artery is generally more anterior and supplies many more branches than the internal carotid artery.

The brachiocephalic and subclavian arteries supply blood to the upper extremities. These are known as inflow arteries. The axillary, brachial, radial, ulnar, palmar, and digital arteries are the intrinsic arteries of the upper extremities and hands. Two digital arteries supply each finger (Fig. 5.10).

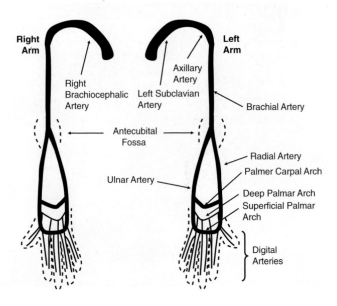

FIGURE 5.10. Depiction of the anatomy of the upper extremities. See text for details.

5.2 Disease Processes

5.2.1 Atherosclerotic Disease

Atherosclerotic disease of the carotid and upper extremities share the same risk factors as atherosclerotic coronary artery disease. However, stroke does not generally result from plaque rupture but rather from embolism of atherosclerotic debris and from thrombosis.

Figures 5.11–5.25 are computed tomographic (CT) angiographic examples of atherosclerosis of the carotid artery system and the arteries of the upper extremities.

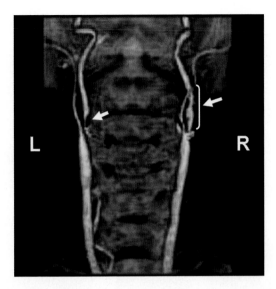

FIGURE 5.11. A volume-rendered, three-dimensional reconstruction, semitransparent image of severe stenoses in proximal segments of both the left and the right internal carotid arteries noted by the *white arrows*. L is left and R is right.

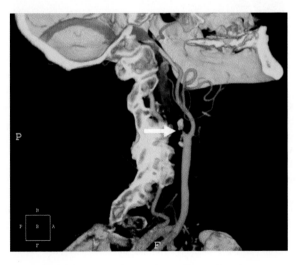

FIGURE 5.12. A volume-rendered, three-dimensional reconstruction of an ostial right internal carotid artery occlusion identified by the *white arrow*.

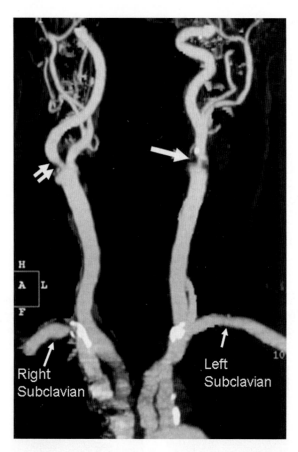

Figure 5.13. Maximum intensity projection (MIP) of a severe distal left common carotid artery stenosis depicted by the *white arrow*. There is also a severe ostial stenosis of the right internal carotid artery demonstrated by the *double white arrows*. Note the nonobstructive calcifications in the proximal left common carotid artery and in both subclavian arteries

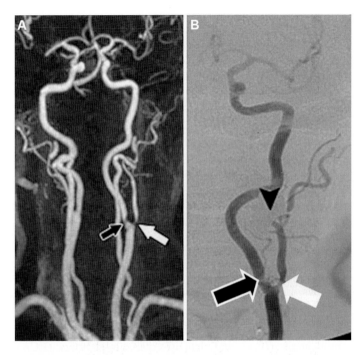

FIGURE 5.14. Panel A is a maximum intensity projection (MIP) of a tight proximal internal carotid artery stenosis (*black arrow*) and a significant ostial external carotid artery stenosis (*white arrow*). Panel B is the corresponding angiogram. Note the occluded external carotid artery branch (*black arrowhead*) not seen on the corresponding CT angiogram.

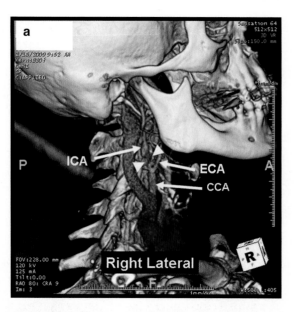

FIGURE 5.15. (**a**) Demonstration of a volume-rendered reconstruction of the right common carotid artery (CCA), right internal carotid artery (ICA), and right external carotid artery (ECA). Between the *arrowheads* is the suggestion of a critical proximal right CCA stenosis. (**b**) A multiplanar reformat (MPR) of the CCA in the same patient depicted in (**a**). Note the identification of a mixed (calcified and noncalcified) stenosis of the proximal right internal carotid artery (between the *arrowheads*). (**c**) Confirmation of the critical right internal carotid artery stenosis suggested by (**a**) and (**b**). This figure represents an axial MPR image demonstrating the critical stenosis (*arrowhead*). Note the small circle of contrast surrounded by low Hounsfield unit plaque and a faint rim of calcium outlining the artery.

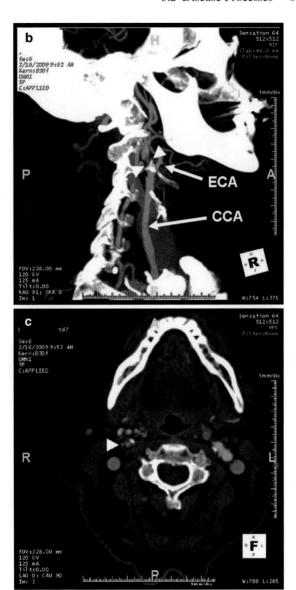

FIGURE 5.15. (continued).

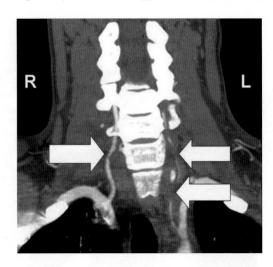

FIGURE 5.16. A coronal, maximum intensity projection (MIP) image demonstrating multiple right and left vertebral artery stenoses (*white arrows*). R is right and L is left.

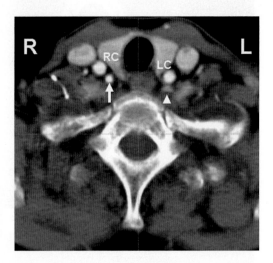

FIGURE 5.17. An axial, maximal intensity projection (MIP) demonstrating a left vertebral artery occlusion (*white arrowhead*). The right vertebral artery is patent (*white arrow*). RC: Right carotid artery. LC: Left carotid artery. R is right and L is left.

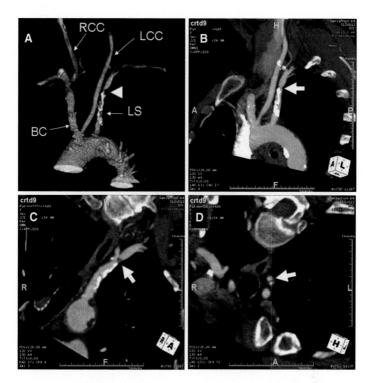

FIGURE 5.18. Depiction of left subclavian artery atherosclerotic disease. Panel A is a volume-rendered image demonstrating the three-dimensional anatomy of this aortic arch and its branch vessels. BC: Brachiocephalic artery. RCC: Right common carotid artery. LCC: Left common carotid artery. LS: Left subclavian artery. Calcific atherosclerotic disease is noted throughout the proximal left subclavian artery with the suggestion of a tight stenosis distal to the calcium marked by the *white arrowhead*. Panel B is a thick maximum intensity projection (MIP) demonstrating similar findings. The multiplanar reformatted (MPR) images confirm the tight stenosis in both the long axis (panel C) and the short axis (panel D).

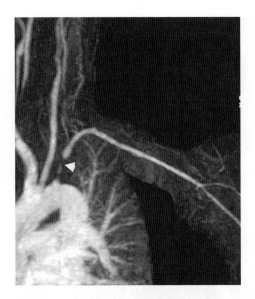

FIGURE 5.19. Depiction of a long proximal and ostial left subclavian artery atherosclerotic stenosis (*white arrowhead*).

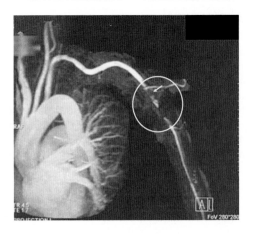

FIGURE 5.20. A left brachial artery embolism (*encircled*). Note the filling defect that suggests a thrombus (*white arrow*).

a

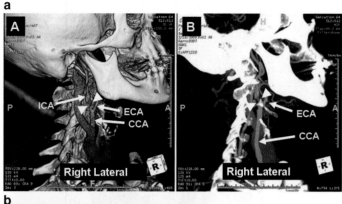

b

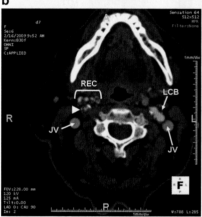

FIGURE 5.21. (**a**) Demonstration of a very severe right internal carotid artery stenosis (between the *white arrowheads* in panels A and B). Panel A is a volume-rendered depiction. Panel B is a maximum intensity projection (MIP). Calcium is noted just prior to the stenosis and is best visualized in panel B. CCA: Right common carotid artery. ICA: Right internal carotid artery. ECA: Right external carotid artery. (**b**) An axial multiplanar reformat (MPR) from the same patient depicted in (**a**). The severe right internal carotid artery stenosis is marked by the *white arrowhead*. REC: Right external carotid artery and branches. LCB: Left carotid artery bifurcation. JV: Jugular veins.

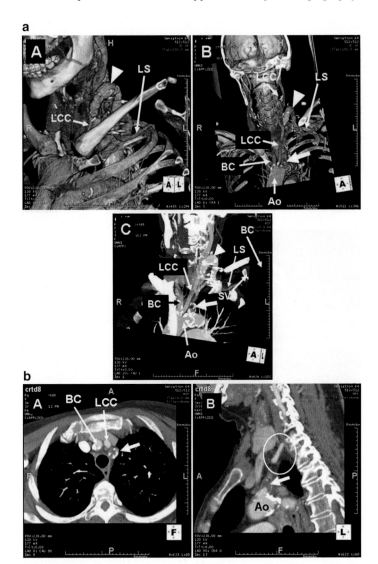

FIGURE 5.22. (**a**) Illustration of an occluded left subclavian artery near the ostium (*white arrow* in panels A, B and C). Panels A and B are volume-rendered depictions demonstrating a graft from the left internal carotid artery to the left subclavian artery (*white arrowhead*). Panel C is a maximum intensity projection of the same. LCC: Left common carotid artery. LS: Left subclavian artery. BC: Brachiocephalic artery. Ao: Aorta. (**b**) The occlusion of the left subclavian artery (*thick white arrow* in panels A and B). The circled artery in panel B is the most distal left subclavian filling via the bypass graft depicted in (**a**). Ao: Aorta. (**c**) Demonstration of a segmented, volume-rendered reconstruction of the anatomy from the patient in (**a**) and (**b**). The graft from the left common carotid artery (LCC) is noted by the *arrowhead*. Both antegrade and retrograde flow are noted in the distal left subclavian artery. LSR: Left subclavian artery retrograde. LSA: Left subclavian artery antegrade. The left vertebral artery (LV) is noted coming off of the left subclavian artery proximal to the distal graft anastomosis. This vessel is filling retrograde. Ao: aorta. BC: Brachiocephalic trunk. RS: Right subclavian artery. RCC: Right common carotid artery. The *thick white arrow* depicts the stump of the left subclavian artery. (**d**) Demonstration of the proximal and distal anastomoses of the bypass graft from the patient depicted in (**a**)–(**c**) (*black arrow* in panel A and *white arrow* in panel B, respectively). Panel A depicts the proximal anastomosis of the bypass graft to the common carotid artery (*black arrow*) and panel B shows the distal anastomosis of the graft to the left subclavian artery (*white arrow*).

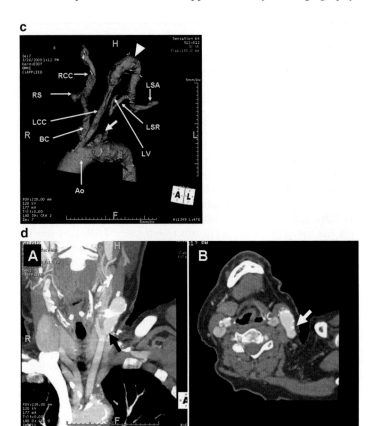

FIGURE 5.22. (continued).

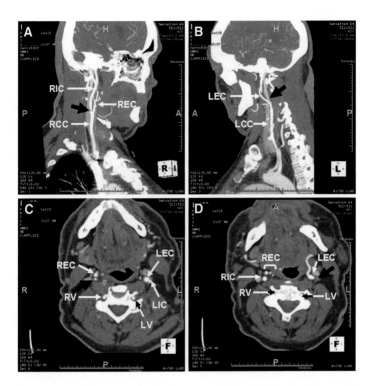

FIGURE 5.23. Panels A–D depict an occluded left internal carotid artery and a severe ostial right internal carotid artery stenosis. Panel A is a maximum intensity projection (MIP) demonstrating the critical ostial right internal carotid artery plaque (*black arrow*). Panel B is an MIP showing the occluded left internal carotid artery (*black arrow*). The internal carotid artery distal to the bifurcation shows no contrast. Panel C is a multiplanar reformat (MPR) in the axial plane. Here the critical right internal carotid artery stenosis is depicted by the *black arrow* just after the bifurcation. The left carotid system is depicted here in an imaging plane proximal to the internal carotid artery occlusion point. Panel D is an MPR at the level of the left internal carotid artery occlusion (a more cranial axial plane than panel C).

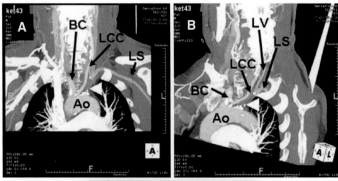

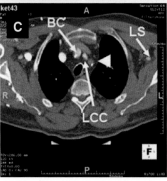

FIGURE 5.24. Illustration of an ostial occlusion of the left subclavian artery with collateralization of the left subclavian artery more distally via the left vertebral artery. Panel A is a maximum intensity projection (MIP) in the coronal plane. The occluded left subclavian stump is marked by the *white arrowhead*. The left subclavian artery (LS) is shown to fill via collaterals. Panel B clearly depicts the left vertebral artery (LV) collateralizing the left subclavian artery. Panel C is a multiplanar reformat (MPR) in the axial plane demonstrating the occluded left subclavian artery (*white arrowhead*) and the LS in short axis filling distally. BC: Brachiocephalic artery. LCC: Left common carotid artery. Ao: Aorta.

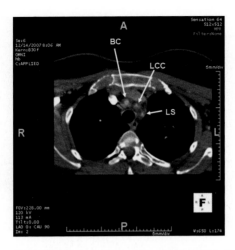

FIGURE 5.25. Illustration of a multiplanar reformat (MPR) in the axial plane at the level just distal to the branch point of the brachio-cephalic artery (BC), the left common carotid artery (LCC), and the left subclavian artery (LS). Note the severe stenoses of the LCC and the LS. The brachiocephalic artery has a more modest stenosis. A rim of noncalcified plaque is noted circumferentially around all three major arch vessels.

Noninvasive detection and accurate quantification of carotid stenoses is clinically very important since detection of carotid disease portends valuable prognostic information regardless of symptoms. Identification of a carotid plaque regardless of the presence of symptoms is a negative predictor of outcome. The 5-year risk of stroke or death in the Asymptomatic Carotid Surgery Trial (ACST)[2] and in the Asymptomatic Carotid Atherosclerosis Trial (ACAS)[3] was 11.8% and 17.5% respectively. The risk of carotid endarterectomy (CEA) was 6.5% in the ACST[2] and 12.4% in the ACAS trial.[3]

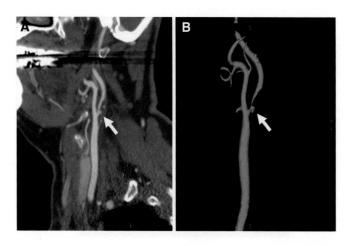

FIGURE 5.26. Depiction of an internal carotid artery ulcerated plaque (*white arrows* in panels A and B). Panel A is a sagittal maximum intensity projection (MIP) and panel B is the corresponding volume-rendered three-dimensional reconstruction.

In addition to accurate quantification of plaque severity, plaque characterization such as the presence or absence of plaque ulceration (Fig. 5.26) has also been shown to be important. Eliasziw et al.[4] found that if a carotid stenosis was symptomatic, the risk of stroke with carotid ulceration medically treated was 26.3% for stenosis graded at 75% and 73.2% if the stenosis was 95%. If no ulcer was present the risk of stroke fell to 21.3% for a 75% stenosis and to 21.3% for a 95% stenosis. Therefore, plaque characterization is an important predictor of future adverse outcomes when assessing carotid atherosclerosis.

As an aside, major venous pathology may also be evaluated and identified by CT angiography (Figs. 5.27–5.29). In addition, ancillary findings may also be found. Figure 5.30 depicts a carotid body tumor and Fig. 5.31 demonstrates an intracranial stimulator used to treat depression.

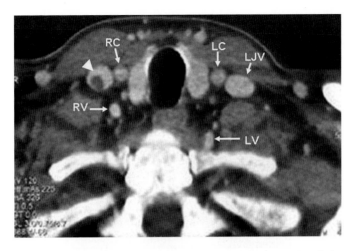

FIGURE 5.27. Demonstration of a right jugular venous thrombus (*white arrowhead*). RV: Right vertebral artery. RC: Right carotid artery. LC: Left carotid artery. LJV: Left jugular vein. LV: Left vertebral artery.

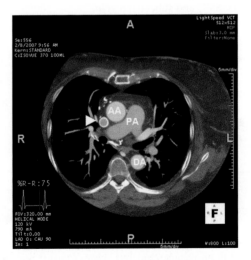

FIGURE 5.28. Illustration of a superior vena cava (SVC) stent (*white arrowhead*) placed in a previously occluded SVC. AA: Ascending aorta. PA: Pulmonary artery. DA: Descending aorta.

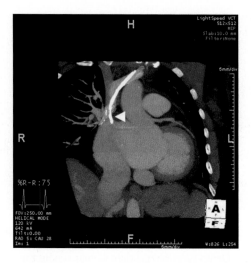

FIGURE 5.29. Depiction of a near occlusion of the superior vena cava (SVC) (*white arrowhead*) at the junction of the SVC and right atrium caused by a pacemaker wire seen as a bright, linear density traversing the SVC and subclavian vein.

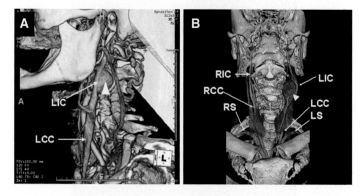

FIGURE 5.30. Illustration of a left carotid body tumor (*white arrowhead*). Panels A and B are volume-rendered images. Panel C is a lateral plane, maximum intensity projection (MIP). Panel D is an axial MIP. RCC: Right common carotid artery. RIC: Right internal carotid artery. RS: Right subclavian artery. LEC: Left external carotid artery. LCC: Left common carotid artery. LIC: Left internal carotid artery. LS: Left subclavian artery.

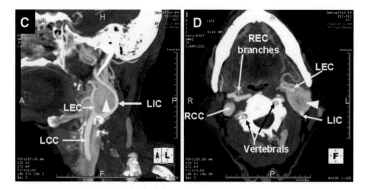

FIGURE 5.30. (continued).

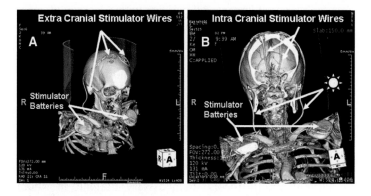

FIGURE 5.31. Depiction of an intracranial stimulator used to treat depression. Panel A is a volume-rendered reconstruction illustrating the stimulator batteries (appear like pacemaker generators) and the extracranial wires traversing the subcutaneous space and curled on top of the cranium. Panel B is a volume-rendered image where the cranium has been cut away demonstrating the stimulator wires traversing the cranial vault and entering the intracranial space. Panel C is a sagittal plane maximal intensity projection (MIP) demonstrating one of the stimulator wires traversing the cranium and entering the brain tissue. Panel D depicts a frontal plane MIP of the same.

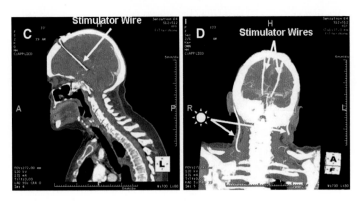

FIGURE 5.31. (continued).

5.2.1.1 Screening and Surveillance

Appropriate screening practices for carotid disease have become standard of care. All patients with a history of coronary bypass surgery, transient ischemic attack, left main coronary artery disease, symptomatic peripheral vascular disease, carotid bruit, and previous carotid surgery should be screened with carotid duplex sonography. Since significant renal artery disease is strongly associated with carotid artery disease, all patients with renal artery stenosis should undergo a carotid duplex examination as well. Finally, patients who have received radiotherapy to the head and neck should be screened beginning 10 years after treatment.[5]

Once carotid artery disease is detected appropriate follow-up surveillance protocols are necessary. Patients in whom carotid stenoses of 20–49% are found should undergo yearly surveillance carotid duplex examinations. In those with stenoses of 50–69% carotid sonograms every 6 months are appropriate. Those who have undergone CEA require ultrasound examinations at 6 weeks, 6 months, 12 months, and annually thereafter. A similar surveillance protocol is followed after carotid stenting.[5]

5.2.1.2 Guidelines for Carotid Endarterectomy[6]

Asymptomatic Patients

Two proven indications are recommended for asymptomatic patients in whom the surgical risk is predicted to be less than 3% and the expected life expectancy is greater than 5 years. The first is an ipsilateral CEA for stenoses greater than or equal to 60% with or without ulceration. The second is a unilateral CEA simultaneous with coronary artery bypass grafting (CABG) for stenosis greater than or equal to 60% with or without ulceration. For those with a stenosis greater than or equal to 50% with ulceration, the benefit of ipsilateral CEA is not proven.

Acceptable but unproven indications include CEA for stenoses greater or equal to 75% with or without ulceration in the presence of a contralateral internal carotid artery stenosis ranging from 75% to 100%. The following indications are uncertain: ipsilateral CEA for a stenosis greater than or equal to 75% with or without ulceration regardless of contralateral carotid, CABG with bilateral asymptomatic carotid stenoses greater than 70% or unilateral CEA with CABG.

Indications that have been proven inappropriate are stenoses less than or equal to 50% with or without ulceration, or ipsilateral CEA for stenoses greater than or equal to 75% irrespective of the contralateral carotid. For patients in whom the expected surgical risk is above 3–5%, there are no proven indications. These patients may be considered for carotid stenting.

Symptomatic Patients

Acceptable indications for CEA include a recent nondisabling event with ipsilateral carotid stenoses greater than 50%. There are no indications proven beneficial for symptomatic patients whose stenoses are less than 50%.

5.2.1.3 Guidelines for Carotid Stenting[6]

Indications for which carotid stenting would currently be favored over CEA include only those anatomic and clinical considerations where CEA is unfavorable. Anatomic issues favoring stenting are prior ipsilateral endarterectomy, contralateral total occlusion, prior irradiation, surgical inaccessibility, contralateral laryngeal palsy, and tracheostomy. In addition, stenting is favored if the patient is a poor surgical candidate.

Considerations when evaluating a carotid stenting candidate include the tortuosity of the carotid vessels, the aortic arch classification (Fig. 5.32), the extent and location of aortic arch atherosclerosis, a string sign greater than 2 cm long, the degree and location of calcium, and the presence or absence of thrombus.

When reading a CT angiogram of the carotid arteries, significant tortuosity and the degree of calcification of the carotid arteries should be noted. Vessel tortuosity may lead to difficulty in placing the stent. Heavy calcium in the carotid artery mandates higher balloon inflation pressures and may lead to bradycardia, especially if the lesion is near the carotid sinus. In addition, some stents are self-expanding and do not have significant radial strength to crack calcium.

Furthermore, straight carotid arterial segments are needed distal to the lesion of interest since embolic protection devices are mandatory and require a 25-mm straight segment landing zone distal to the lesion. Vertebral stenting is also feasible with a distal embolic protection device in place. The arch type is important in predicting the ease of accessing the carotids with the guiding catheter and wire. Type 2 and 3 arches are technically more difficult for carotid stenting.

The risk for carotid stent restenosis is 2.5–5%.[7] The usual treatment for in-stent restenosis is balloon angioplasty. Results of carotid stenting are currently based on small studies in high-risk surgical candidates. The largest study so far

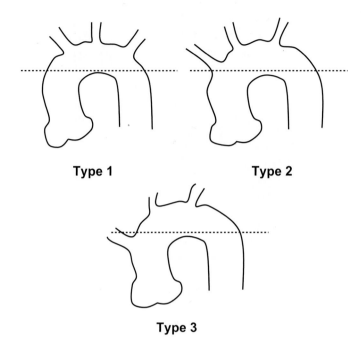

Type 1   **Type 2**

Type 3

FIGURE 5.32. A cartoon demonstrating the classification system for the aortic arch. Type 1 describes the three great vessels arising well above the imaginary line drawn across the lesser curvature of the arch. Type 2 occurs when the right brachiocephalic artery arises at the line drawn parallel to the lesser curvature of the arch. Finally, Type 3 is when the right brachiocephalic artery arises well below the lesser curvature line. Types 2 and 3 are technically more difficult to engage when attempting carotid artery stenting.

was that of Roubin et al.[7] who published a 30-day fatal stroke rate of 0.6% and a nonstroke death rate of 1%. He found the major and minor stroke rates to be 1% and 4.8% respectively. The overall combined stroke and death rate was 7.4%. Over 5 years, the stroke rate after 30 days was 3.2%.

Figure 5.33 demonstrates bilateral carotid stents.

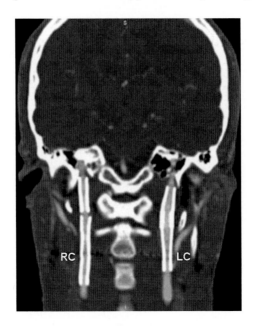

FIGURE 5.33. Demonstration of multiple stents in both the right internal carotid (RC) and the left internal carotid (LC) arteries.

5.2.2 Aneurysms

Aneurysms of the carotid, vertebral, subclavian, and axillary arteries are rare. Subclavian artery aneurysms usually result from atherosclerosis, trauma, thoracic outlet syndrome, and rarely from collagen vascular diseases. Axillary artery aneurysms result mainly from trauma. Since aneurysms in these arteries are unusual, finding an aneurysms in these locations should prompt a search for aneurysms in other locations. Figures 5.34–5.36 depict carotid, vertebral, and subclavian artery aneurysms respectively.

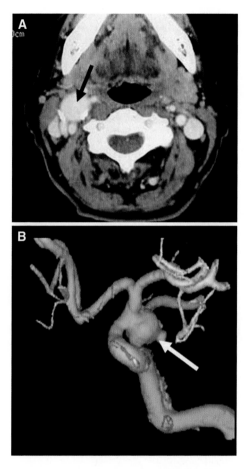

FIGURE 5.34. Panel A illustrates a maximum intensity projection (MIP) in the axial plane of a right internal carotid artery aneurysm (*black arrow*). Panel B demonstrates the aneurysm in a segmented, volume-rendered reconstruction (*white arrow*).

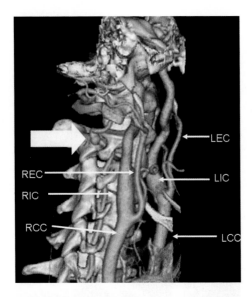

FIGURE 5.35. A right vertebral artery aneurysm (*block arrow*). REC: Right external carotid artery. RIC: Right internal carotid artery. RCC: Right common carotid artery. LEC: Left external carotid artery. LIC: Left internal carotid artery. LCC: Left common carotid artery.

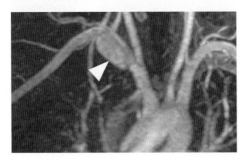

FIGURE 5.36. A segmented, thick maximum intensity projection (MIP) of a right subclavian fusiform aneurysm (*arrowhead*). The MIP thickness was intentionally increased to demonstrate the entire anatomy.

5.2.3 Thoracic Outlet Syndrome

Thoracic outlet syndrome occurs when there is obstruction of the neurovascular bundle as it exits the thoraco-cervical region and passes to the axilla. The arterial and nerve bundles must pass between the scalene muscles, through the space bordered by the clavicle, the first rib, and scapula, and under the pectoralis minor muscle. All three of these areas may potentially compress the neurovascular bundle and lead to symptoms. Often these potential compression sites are occupied by congenital anomalies such as cervical ribs and fibrous bands that may induce positional compression of nerves and blood vessels. Congenital, traumatic, or age-related muscle weakness and sagging may induce the syndrome as well.

Often numbness, weakness, and a sensation of swelling of the upper limbs suggest thoracic outlet syndrome. The initial clinical presentation depends on whether the nerves or the blood vessels are the predominant point of compression.[8] Pure vascular obstruction is rare and may induce color changes, swelling, or diffuse forearm and hand pain.[8] Pure neurologic compression is also rare and may lead to loss of sensation and muscle atrophy.[8] More commonly, there is an overlap of vascular and neural symptoms.[8] It is possible that in the latter group, no physical findings are present. Intermittent paresthesias may also occur in these latter patients. Patients may also experience an aching in the shoulder or arm.

If the diagnosis of thoracic outlet syndrome is suspected, provocative physical exam testing is then necessary. Other studies may be necessary when the diagnosis is less clear, when initial attempts at conservative treatment fail, or when severe symptoms are present.

Many provocative tests have been described and are discussed below. The sensitivity and specificity of these tests are relatively low (between 46% and 62%).[9, 10] These tests are helpful if they result in a diminished pulse or if they reproduce symptoms.

The Roos test is when the patient repeatedly clenches and unclenches the fists while keeping the arms abducted and externally rotated (palms forward and upward).[11]

The modified Adson test serves to evaluate whether tension in the scalene muscles causes compression of the neurovascular bundle. With the patient seated and arms at his or her side, the radial pulse is palpated at the wrist and auscultation is performed in the supra-clavicular space. The patient then performs a Valsalva maneuver with the neck fully extended, the affected arm elevated, and the chin turned away from the involved side. A positive test results in a diminished pulsation of the radial artery and a bruit over the axillary vessels. The patient may also become aware of increased paresthesias.[12]

The hyperabduction maneuver tests whether constriction of the neurovascular bundle occurs beneath the insertion of the pectoralis minor tendon into the coracoid process. The patient raises his or her hands above the head with the elbows partially flexed and extending out laterally from the body. A decrease in radial pulse and reproduction of symptoms are suggestive of the diagnosis.

The costo-clavicular maneuver is performed by having the patient take an exaggerated military position of attention with the shoulders thrust backward and downward. This maneuver tests for compression between the ribs and the clavicles. A positive test is marked by features similar to a positive modified Adson test. These findings include a decreased radial pulse, a diminished pulse amplitude or bruit in the costo-clavicular space, and paresthesias.

Imaging studies may also be performed to evaluate for thoracic outlet syndrome. Cervical spine plane films or a chest x-ray may identify a cervical rib or an elongated C7 transverse process. These findings may be helpful but are not specific since they may be present without symptoms and since the syndrome may occur in the absence of these findings.

Doppler studies have improved with more advanced technology and may be used instead of more invasive testing in patients with physical findings of vascular compression or obstruction. CT angiography or magnetic resonance angiography (MRA) may be performed in patients with a predominantly vascular presentation. Nerve conduction studies may be useful in neurological presentations to confirm nerve entrapment and identify the location of the entrapment.

Conservative management is most often the best and should be pursued unless serious symptoms are present. Fewer than 5% of patients require surgical treatment.[13] In addition, patients should be made aware of the factors that exacerbate compression at the thoracic outlet. Posture correction, keeping the arms down at night and avoiding hyperabduction, should be recommended. Exercises to strengthen the muscles surrounding the thoracic outlet should be emphasized. Particularly useful exercises include neck erector strengthening and shoulder shrugs.

Physical therapy and exercise, instructions in proper sitting, and proper work and sleep positions, may provide relief within 6 weeks. Surgical intervention should be considered when signs of muscle wasting, continuous sensory loss, incapacitating pain, or worsening circulatory impairment are present. Surgical treatment appears to be very successful for relieving the pain and sensory disturbance, but is less effective for muscle weakness.[14]

Figure 5.37a–c depict a nice example of a CT angiography study demonstrating thoracic outlet syndrome.

5.2.4 Raynaud's Phenomenon

Raynaud's phenomenon is characterized by an exaggerated vascular response to cold or emotional distress and may manifest as sharp demarcation of skin color in the digits due to abnormal vasoconstriction of the digital arteries and skin arterioles. A local defect in the normal vascular response is implicated in this disorder.[15] Primary Raynaud's disease occurs when no associated disorder is found. Secondary Raynaud's syndrome is diagnosed when an associated disorder such as a collagen vascular disease is present.

The prevalence of this disease ranges from 5% to 20% in women and 4% to 14% in men.[16] Raynaud's disease is more common in women and younger patients. It is also more prevalent in patients with a family history of the phenomenon.[17]

Most often, Raynaud's disease affects the hands, though the toes may frequently be involved. Typically, an attack is characterized by a sudden feeling of cold fingers or toes in response to sudden and possibly mild decreases in temperature or with sudden activation of the sympathetic nervous system such as with emotional stress. A key distinguishing point is the sharply demarcated color difference in the digits, which either turn white or blue. With warming of the digits or relief of the emotional stressor, the skin will return to normal in about 20 min. The attack often begins in a single finger and spreads from there with the thumb often being spared. Other places of thermoregulatory vessels may also be involved, such as the ears, nose, face, and knees. Generalized livedo reticularis may also be present. Symptoms of decreased blood flow may include pain, paresthesias, numbness, and clumsiness of the hand or foot.

The diagnosis is predominantly historical as no reliable diagnostic test or maneuver exists. Definite Raynaud's disease includes a history of repeated episodes of biphasic, sharply demarcated color changes when exposed to cold or emotional stress.[18] Possible Raynaud's disease is diagnosed when there is uniphasic, sharply demarcated color changes in addition to numbness or paresthesias upon exposure to cold or emotional stress.[18] Raynaud's syndrome is excluded when there is no color change associated with the symptoms.[18]

FIGURE 5.37. (a) Demonstration of an example of thoracic outlet syndrome diagnosed by computed tomographic (CT) angiography. Panel A is a volume-rendered image of the left subclavian artery (LS), left axial artery (AA), and left brachial artery (BA) with the left arm raised above the head. Kinking is noted distal to the artery's exit from the space between the clavicle and the first rib (*white arrowhead*). This finding is again demonstrated in the maximum intensity projection (MIP) in panel B. (b) Two volume-rendered images from the patient depicted in (a). Again the left arm is raised above the head. No dynamic obstruction is noted as the artery exits the space between the scalene muscles of the neck (panel A, *circled area*). Furthermore, no stenosis is noted as the artery travels between the clavicle and the first rib (panel B, *circled area*). (c) A multiplanar reformat (MPR) demonstrating nicely that the kink in the left subclavian artery from the patient depicted in (a) and (b) is due to compression from a band of muscles located in the axilla (*white arrow* in panels A and B).

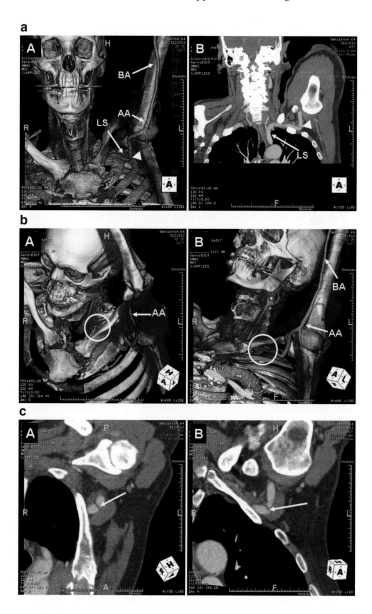

When the diagnosis of Raynaud's phenomenon is made, it is important to rule out secondary causes which may include connective tissue diseases, atherosclerosis, embolic disease, Buerger's disease, drug-induced Raynaud's disease, vibration-induced Raynaud's disease, vascular trauma, and frostbite.

5.2.5 Buerger's Disease

Buerger's disease or thromboangiitis obliterans is a noninflammatory condition usually involving the small arteries and veins of the extremities and progresses proximally as the disease advances. Buerger's disease spares the blood vessel walls. Distinguishing factors from classical vasculitis include a negative sedimentation rate, normal autoantibody tests, and normal circulating antibody tests.[19] The incidence in the United States is 12.6 per 100,000 persons.[20] Men are more commonly affected than women and the usual age of onset is the early to mid-40s.[21] Tobacco abuse is a necessary component of this disease process.[22]

The acute pathophysiology involves the formation of occlusive, inflammatory thrombi in the arteries and veins of the distal extremities. Inflammatory cells may be present in the thrombi. The intermediate phase is characterized by organization of the thrombus, and in the chronic phase, inflammation resolves and organized thrombus and fibrosis persists.[23]

Clinically, the disease usually presents with ischemia of the digits manifesting as claudication of the hands, feet, calves, arms, and thighs in a smoker.[24] Ulcer formation is common. The clinical diagnostic criteria include age less than 45 years, current or recent history of tobacco use, and distal extremity ischemia.[25] A definitive diagnosis is confirmed with histopathology in the acute phase. Certainly, other inflammatory diseases should be excluded and embolic phenomenon should be ruled out. Smoking cessation is the only definitive treatment. Smoking cessation prevents amputation in 94%. In those who continue to smoke, up to 43% will eventually require an amputation.[24]

5.3 Accuracy of Carotid and Upper Extremity CT Angiography

Fortunately, CT angiography of the carotid and upper extremity arteries is a robust and accurate technique with a pooled sensitivity of 95% and a specificity of 98% compared to digital subtraction angiography (DSA).[26] There is a close agreement in stenosis severity and plaque characterization with MRA and DSA.[26] Because of a superior spatial resolution, CT angiography is at least as good as, if not better than, MRA in this arena. Bartlett et al.[27] reported an interobserver correlation of 0.78–0.89 for carotid CT angiography. In his study, the sensitivity for detecting a stenosis of 70% or greater was 88% and the specificity was 92% with a negative predictive value of 98%.[27]

CT angiography has been shown to be comparable to MRA for the detection of ulcerated stenoses and slightly better for detecting irregular stenoses. Since CT angiography may provide a detailed characterization of the plaque itself, it is more advantageous than DSA in plaque evaluation. However, in theory, calcium may hide ulceration and this limitation may hinder CT angiography in evaluating some carotid stenoses.

5.4 Approach to Reading Carotid and Upper Extremity CT Angiography

As with all CT angiograms, we recommend starting with an assessment of the scan quality for contrast opacification and artifacts. Next, a survey of the three-dimensional (3-D) data set is recommended to generally characterize the anatomy and to identify areas that may require more detailed analyses. Diagnoses are never made from the 3-D data alone as these images are prone to error. Once the 3-D data is evaluated, we primarily use axial maximum intensity projection (MIP) images. Sagittal, coronal, and oblique imaging planes may also be helpful. Curved multiplanar reformatted (MPR) images are employed to further analyze difficult arterial segments. Ultimately, the stenoses degree and character are best assessed and confirmed with MPR images.

We recommend that the physician characterizes the atherosclerotic burden, the vessel tortuosity, the arch classification, the extent of and location of calcium, and the stenosis degree. Unlike with coronary arteries, when a carotid artery lumen is completely obscured by calcium an underlying tight stenosis is often present. After analyzing the carotids, the vertebral arteries should be assessed. Since parts of the vertebral arteries reside within the spinal foramen, the lumen may be obscured by bone. The cerebral arteries should be followed as best as possible through the cranium where brain aneurysms may be identified. Finally, the visualized portions of the subclavian arteries should be analyzed.

Chapter 6
Thoracic Aortic CT Angiography

6.1 Anatomy

The thoracic aorta extends from aortic annulus to the diaphragm and includes the ascending aorta, the aortic arch, and the descending thoracic aorta. The first 3 cm of the proximal aorta are intrapericardial. The thoracic aorta anatomy may be seen in Figs. 5.1–5.3.

The ascending aorta is comprised of the aortic root and the tubular portion. The aortic root is made up of the right, left, and noncoronary sinuses of Valsalva. The right and left coronary arteries are the only normal branches of the ascending aorta. The tubular portion of the ascending aorta extends from the sino-tubular junction to the brachiocephalic trunk. The normal diameter of aortic root is≤3.9 cm. Smaller sizes are considered normal in smaller persons. The normal tubular diameter is ≤3.5 cm at the level of the right pulmonary artery.

The aortic arch extends from the brachiocephalic trunk to the origin of the left subclavian artery and is followed by the isthmus which extends to the attachment of the ligamentum arteriosum (often and normally calcified). The diameter of the normal aortic arch is ≤3 cm. There are usually three branches of the aortic arch. These branches in order from proximal to distal include the brachiocephalic trunk (innominate artery), the left common carotid artery, and the left subclavian artery.

R. Pelberg and W. Mazur, *Vascular CT Angiography Manual*, 91
DOI: 10.1007/978-1-84996-260-5_6,

A complete listing of the normal published thoracic aortic diameters are noted in Table 6.1.[28] Table 6.2 demonstrates the gender differences in aortic root and ascending aortic measurements.[28]

Normal variant aortic arches include the bovine arch (common ostium for the innominate and right carotid arteries, Fig. 5.5) and the left vertebral artery arising from the

TABLE 6.1 Published normal adult thoracic aorta diameters at multiple levels[28]

Adult thoracic aorta diameter	
Category	Diameter (cm)
Female root	3.50–3.72
Male root	3.63–3.91
Ascending (male and female)	2.86
Female mid descending	2.54–2.64
Male mid descending	2.29–2.98
Female diaphragm level	2.40–2.44
Male diaphragm level	2.43–2.69

TABLE 6.2 Normal gender differences in adult ascending aorta dimensions[28]

	Gender differences in adult aortic root dimensions			
	Men		Woman	
	Absolute (cm)	Indexed (cm/m²)	Absolute (cm)	Indexed (cm/m²)
Annulus	2.6 ± 0.3	1.3 ± 0.1	2.3 ± 0.2	1.3 ± 0.1
Sinuses of Valsalva	3.4 ± 0.3	1.7 ± 0.2	3.0 ± 0.3	1.8 ± 0.2
Sinotubular junction	2.9 ± 0.3	1.5 ± 0.2	2.6 ± 0.3	1.5 ± 0.2
Proximal ascending aorta	3.0 ± 0.4	1.5 ± 0.2	2.7 ± 0.4	1.6 ± 0.3

aortic arch itself (Fig. 5.6). The term bovine aortic arch is a misnomer since cattle actually have a common brachiocephalic trunk arising from the arch and splitting into two subclavian arteries from which the neck vessels arise.

Another common aortic arch variant is the ductus diverticulum (Fig. 6.1). A ductus diverticulum is a developmental

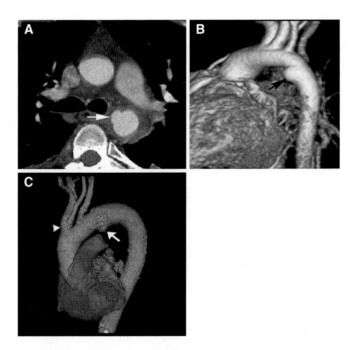

Fig. 6.1 Illustration of two examples of a ductus diverticulum depicted by the *white arrows* in panels A and C and the *black arrow* in panel B. Panels A and B are from one patient and panel C is from a separate patient. Note the location on the inner curvature of the aortic arch and the smoothness of the out pouching. In addition, the angles are obtuse. The *white arrowhead* in panel C marks the common trunk of the bracheocephalic artery and left common carotid artery (bovine arch). (Reproduced with kind permission from Elsevier. Copyright 2007. Abbara S, Kalva S, Cury RC, et al. Thoracic aortic disease: spectrum of multidetector computed tomography imaging findings. *J Cardiovasc Comput Tomogr.* 2007;1(1):43)

out pouching of the aorta which is usually seen at the antero-medial aspect of the aorta at the site of the previous ductus arteriosus. It appears as a focal bulge along the inner curvature of the isthmus and may be confused with a pseudoaneurysm (Figs. 6.2 and 6.3) or penetrating ulcer (Fig. 6.4). The ductus diverticulum is usually smooth with obtuse angles, whereas a pseudoaneurysm or penetrating ulcer usually demonstrates acute angles. In addition, the ductus diverticulum is usually located on the inner curvature of the aorta. A pseudoaneurysm or penetrating ulcer may be located anywhere along the aorta.

The descending thoracic aorta extends from the isthmus to the diaphragm. The normal diameter is ≤2.5 cm (tables 6-1 and 6-2) Descending thoracic aortic branches include bronchial, spinal, intercostal, and the superior phrenic arteries as well as various mediastinal branches.

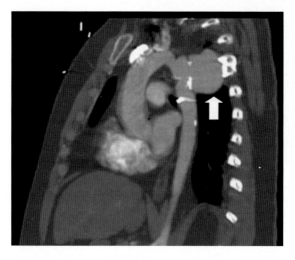

Fig. 6.2 Illustration of a descending aorta pseudoaneurysm (*white arrow*). Note the narrow neck and the acute angles with the aorta

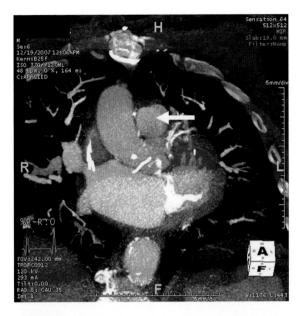

Fig. 6.3 Another example of a pseudoaneurysm (*white arrow*) resulting from valve replacement surgery

6.2 Disease Processes

Aortic disease may span the entire aorta or may be multifocal. Clinical presentations range from asymptomatic with clinically undetectable thoracic aortic aneurysms to symptoms of severe chest pain from acute aortic dissection. Atypical presentations of these common pathologies are frequent and aortic disease often remains undetected until a life-threatening complication occurs or until detected serendipitously on imaging studies performed for other purposes. Since the treatment results for most stable, potentially asymptomatic, possibly high-risk thoracic aorta diseases is

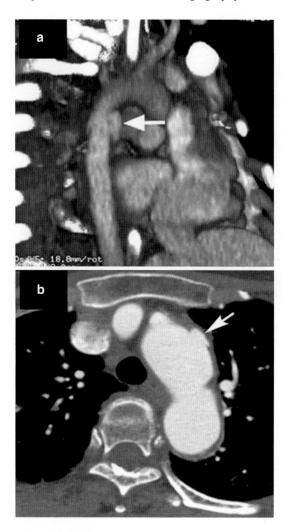

Fig. 6.4 Illustration of a penetrating aortic ulcer (*white arrows*). Panel A is an oblique plane, black and white, thick maximum intensity projection (MIP). Panel B is an MIP in the axial plane. Of note, the angles of the ulcer with the aorta are sharp or acute in contrast to the obtuse angles of the ductus diverticulum. (Reproduced with kind permission from Elsevier. Copyright 2007. Abbara S, Kalva S, Cury RC, et al. Thoracic aortic disease: spectrum of multi-detector computed tomography imaging findings. *J Cardiovasc Comput Tomogr.* 2007;1(1):43–54)

more favorable than for acute presentations of thoracic vascular catastrophes, early identification of these disease states is essential.

6.2.1 Thoracic Aortic Atherosclerosis

Atherosclerosis of the aorta is a common disease entity with similar risks as those for coronary atherosclerosis including age, hypertension, smoking, diabetes, hyperlipidemia, and family history of atherosclerosis. Atherosclerotic disease of the aorta is associated with many of the disease entities listed in this chapter.

The histological classifications of atherosclerotic lesions are described here.[29] Type 1 lesions are the earliest atherosclerotic lesions containing only macrophages and foam cells. Type II lesions or the fatty streak contains mostly intracellular lipids. Type III or intermediate lesions contain small extracellular lipids pools. Type IV lesions are called atheromas and consist of type II lesions with a large core of extracellular lipids. Type V lesions are termed fibroatheromas and these lesions contain a lipid core and a fibrotic layer. There may also be multiple lipid cores and fibrotic layers. These may be calcific or fibrotic only. Type VI or complicated lesions may have a defect on the lesion surface or may demonstrate hemorrhage, hematoma, or thrombus in the plaque.

6.2.2 Thoracic Aortic Aneurysm

An aortic aneurysm is defined as a focal dilation of greater than 50% of the normal diameter of the aorta.

A pseudoaneurysm (false aneurysm) represents a disruption of the arterial wall with extravasation of blood contained only by the periarterial connective tissue and not by the arterial wall itself. Ectasia is defined as arterial dilation that reaches a size less than 50% greater than the normal arterial diameter. Arteriomegaly represents diffuse arterial dilation (of greater than 50% relative to the normal segment)involving multiple portions of an artery. Thoracic aortic aneurysms involve the portion of the aorta above the diaphragm and thoracoabdominal aortic aneurysms are aneurysms that involve both the thoracic aorta and abdominal aorta (below the diaphragm). Aortic dissection is a disruption of the intimal layer of the aorta with bleeding between the intima and the media and adventitia.

The intima represents the endothelial layer of the aorta that rests on the basement membrane. The intima has minimal connective tissue. The media is contained within the internal elastic lamina and is formed mainly by smooth muscle cells. The adventitia represents a tough layer of collagen and contains the vasa vasorum and the arterial nerves. Vasa vasorum can traverse the outer portion of the media as well.

The incidence of thoracic aortic aneurysms is estimated to be around six cases per 100,000 patient years.[30] Less common than abdominal aortic aneurysms, they occur most commonly in the sixth and seventh decade of life.[30] Males are affected approximately 2–4 times more commonly than females.[30] Hypertension is a comorbid condition in over 60% of patients.[30] Up to 13% of patients diagnosed with an aortic aneurysm are found to have multiple aneurysms and approximately 20–25% of patients with large thoracic aortic aneurysm also have an abdominal aortic aneurysm.[31]

Four general anatomic categories of thoracic aortic aneurysms have been described and include the ascending aorta, the aortic arch, the descending aorta, and the thoracoabdominal aorta.[30] Ascending aortic aneurysms arise anywhere from the aortic valve to the innominate artery and represent 60% of all thoracic aortic aneurysms.[30] Aortic arch aneurysms include any thoracic aneurysm that involves the brachiocephalic vessels and represent 10% of all thoracic aortic aneurysms.[30] Descending aortic aneurysms arise distal to the left subclavian artery and comprise 40% of these aneurysms.[30] Finally, thoraco-abdominal aneurysms involve both the thoracic and abdominal aorta and represent 10% of all thoracic aortic aneurysms.[30]

Ascending thoracic aortic aneurysms most often result from cystic medial degeneration that leads to weakening of the aortic wall.[32] Cystic medial degeneration occurs normally with aging and is more prevalent and accelerated in patients with hypertension. Marfan's syndrome is the most common cause of cystic medial degeneration in young patients. Other less common connective tissue disorders such as Ehlers–Danlos syndrome are also associated with cystic medial degeneration.

Isolated sinus of Valsalva aneurysms (Fig. 6.5) can occur and are located most commonly in the right sinus followed by the noncoronary sinus.[33] Aneurysms of the left sinus of Valsalva are rare.[33] Surgical correction for sinus of Valsalva aneurysms is controversial because their natural history is not clear. Treatment is indicated if significant aortic insufficiency is present, symptoms of compression occur, or if rupture ensues. Generally, the outcomes of surgical corrective procedures are excellent, especially if the surgical risk of the patient is acceptable.

Aneurysms of the aortic root (Fig. 6.6) appear as an efface-ment of the sino-tubular junction (pear-shaped aorta). Root aneurysms are most closely associated with Marfan's, bicus-pid aortic valve, Ehlers–Danlos syndrome, and familial thoracic aortic aneurysm syndromes.[33]

Aneurysms of the tubular ascending aorta (Fig. 6.7) are mostly idiopathic, but may also be associated with bicuspid aortic valve, atherosclerotic disease, giant cell arteritis, syphilis (rare in the present), or familial thoracic aneurysm syndromes.[33]

Descending thoracic aneurysms (Fig. 6.8) are most often associated with atherosclerosis and the risk factors for aneurysm formation are the same as those for atherosclerosis.[32] However, it remains unclear whether atherosclerosis itself is the actual cause of aneurysm formation.[34] It seems likely that there may be a systemic, nonatherosclerotic process at work,

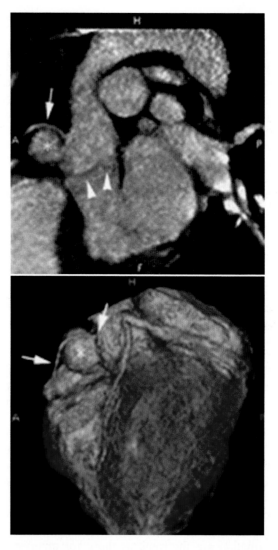

Fig. 6.5 An example of a sinus of Valsalva aneurysm (*white arrows*) seen in maximum intensity projection format (*upper panel*) and in 3-D reformatting (*lower panel*). The *arrow heads* in the upper panels represent the two of the three coronary sinuses. (Reproduced with kind permission of Springer Science + Business Media. Kuo K-H, Tiu C-M. Coronary CT angiography with reformatting demonstrates a sinus of Valsalva aneurysm. *Pedeatr Radiol.* 2008;38:1262)

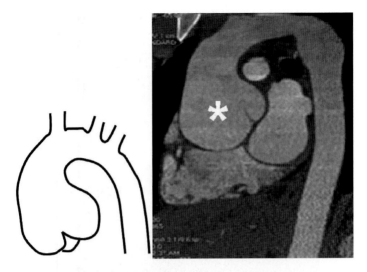

Fig. 6.6 Demonstration of an aortic root aneurysm (*white asterisk*) in both cartoon format and by computed tomographic angiography. Note the effacement of the sino-tubular junction and the so-called pear-shaped aorta

such as a defect in vascular structural proteins, with atherosclerosis occurring secondarily.[35]

Most theories emphasize the primary role of protein and collagen breakdown within the extracellular matrix by proteases such as collagenase, elastase, various matrix metalloproteinases, and plasmin. Proteolytic factors are derived from endothelial and smooth muscle cells and from inflammatory cells infiltrating the media and adventitia.[36] But the combination of protein degradation and mechanical factors are thought to cause the cystic medial necrosis necessary for aneurysm formation. Cystic medial necrosis has the appearance of smooth muscle cell necrosis and elastic fiber degeneration with cystic spaces filled with mucoid material. These changes result in vessel dilatation and subsequent aneurysm formation and possible rupture.

Bicuspid aortic valve (even in the absence of significant valvular stenosis or regurgitation), Marfan's syndrome, and

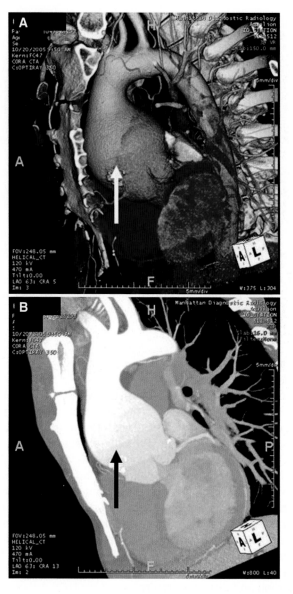

Fig. 6.7 Representation of a tubular ascending aortic aneurysm in 3-D (Panel A) and maximum intensity projection (Panel B) demonstrated by the *white* and *black arrows*, respectively. Note that the aneurysm mostly spares the sinuses of Valsalva

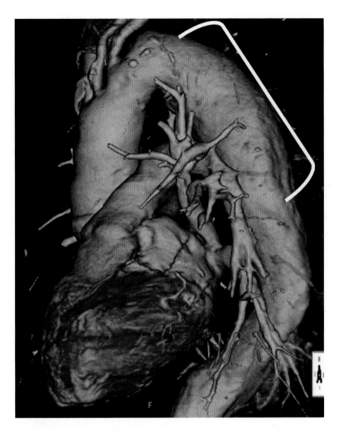

Fig. 6.8 Three-dimensional depiction of a fusiform descending thoracic aortic aneurysm. The ascending aorta is also dilated but the aortic arch is spared. The ascending aorta is also mildly dilated

Ehlers–Danlos syndrome are also associated with tubular aortic aneurysm formation.

In Marfan's syndrome, aortic root disease is the main cause of morbidity and mortality.[37] Cystic medial degeneration often precedes aneurysm formation.[38] Echocardiography demonstrates dilation of the aortic root in 60–80% of adult patients with Marfan's.[39] Fifty percent of children will have aortic root dilation as well. Marfan's pathology may also involve other segments of the thoracic aorta, the abdominal aorta, or even the carotid and intracranial arteries.[40] Type I dissections may result if these patients are not treated appropriately. Dissections in Marfan's patients typically begin just above the coronary ostia (Debakey Type I) and may extend to the entire length of the diseased aorta. Approximately 10% of dissections begin distal to the left subclavian (Debakey type II), but dissection is rarely limited to just the thoracic aorta.[41]

The Ehlers–Danlos syndrome is a group of conditions resulting in defects in type III collagen, which cause hyperelasticity and fragility of the skin and hypermobility of the joints. Mitral valve prolapse is often present. Although aortic root dilatation is uncommon and aortic dissection is rare, spontaneous rupture of large- and medium-sized arteries, usually without dissection, is the most serious cardiovascular complication. A number of mutations have been identified including mutations in the transforming growth factor beta receptor 2 gene which is responsible for about 5% of familial cases.[42]

Other genetic mutations that are associated with thoracic aortic aneurysms and dissections at smaller aortic diameters have been noted as well. The Loeys–Dietz syndrome is newly discovered autosomal dominant genetic disease similar to Marfan syndrome. It is caused by mutations in the genes encoding transforming growth factor beta receptor 1 (TGFBR1) or 2 (TGFBR2). Its characteristics included orbital hypertelorism, cleft palate or bifid uvula and aortic dilation, aneurysms and dissection. The arteries are often tortuous. It may also include scoliosis, pectus excavatum or pectus carinatum, and camptodactyly. Long fingers, club foot, craniosynostosis, joint hypermobility, patent ductus arteriosus, and atrial septal defects are also seen. Arnold–Chiari malformations, translucent skin, and bicuspid aortic valves have been associated as well.

Other associated genetic mutations have been documented to be associated with thoracic aortic disease such as TGFBR1, TGFBR2, FBN1, ACTA2, COL3A1, and MYH11.

Class I recommendations for genetic syndromes include (Table 6.3)[28]: (1) An echocardiogram at the time of diagnosis for Marfan syndrome to assess the aorta and at 6 months to

TABLE 6.3 Class I indications for genetic predisposition syndromes

1. Echocardiogram at the time of diagnosis of Marfan syndrome to assess the aorta and repeated at 6 months to evaluate for rate of change

2. Annual imaging for Marfan patients if stability is noted. More frequent imaging for Marfan patients if the maximal aortic diameter is ≥ 4.5 cm or if growth occurs

3. Complete aortic imaging at diagnosis and at 6 months in Loeys–Dietz syndrome patients or those with other predisposing genetic mutations

4. Yearly magnetic resonance imaging (reduce radiation) from head to pelvis in Loeys–Dietz patients

5. Imaging of the heart and aorta in Turner syndrome patients to exclude bicuspid aortic valve, coarctation, and thoracic aortic disease. If normal, repeat imaging in 5–10 years. If abnormal then yearly imaging

6. Aortic imaging for first-degree relatives of patients with thoracic aortic aneurysm or dissection. If a first-degree relative is positive it is Class IIa to image second-degree relatives

7. Genetic counseling and testing for first-degree relatives of genetic mutation patients. Imaging is recommended if a mutation is found

8. Evaluation for bicuspid aortic valve and asymptomatic thoracic aortic disease in first-degree relatives of patients with bicuspid aortic valve, premature aortic vascular disease, or familial forms of thoracic aortic disease

9. Aortic imaging to exclude coarctation and aortic aneurysm in all bicuspid aortic valve patients

evaluate the rate of change. (2) Annual imaging for Marfan patients if stability is noted. More frequent imaging should be performed if the maximal aortic diameter is greater than or equal to 4.5 cm or if growth occurs. (3) Patients with Loeys–Dietz syndrome or other predisposing genetic mutations should have complete aortic imaging at diagnosis and at 6 months. (4) Loeys Dietz patients should have yearly magnetic resonance imaging from the cerebral circulation to the pelvis. (5) Turner syndrome patients require imaging of the heart and aorta to rule out bicuspid aortic valve, coarctation and thoracic aorta dilation. If normal and no other risk factors, repeat imaging in 5 to 10 years. If abnormalities are found yearly imaging is recommended. (6) Aortic imaging is recommended in first-degree relatives of patients with thoracic aortic aneurysm and/or dissection. (7) First-degree relatives of patients with associated genetic mutations should undergo counseling and testing. If a genetic mutation is found, imaging is recommended. (8) First-degree relatives of patients with bicuspid aortic valve, premature aortic vascular disease, or with the familial form of thoracic aortic disease should be evaluated for the presence of bicuspid aortic valve and asymptomatic thoracic aortic disease. (9) All patients with bicuspid aortic valve should have aortic imaging performed.

Thoracic aneurysms may be fusiform or saccular. Fusiform aneurysms (Fig. 6.9) are uniform in shape with symmetrical dilation that involves the entire circumference of the aortic wall, whereas saccular aneurysms (Fig. 6.10) are more localized and appear as an out pouching of only a portion of the

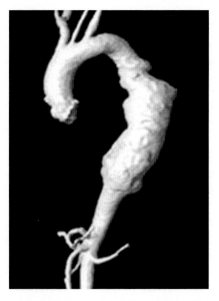

Fig. 6.9 A segmented, volume-rendered CT angiogram of a fusiform descending aortic aneurysm

Saccular Aneurysm

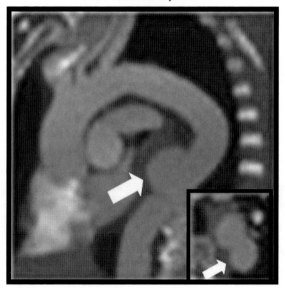

Fig. 6.10 Depiction of a thick maximum intensity projection of a saccular descending aorta aneurysm in long axis (*large white arrow*) and in short axis (*small white arrow* in the lower right box). Note the broad base which distinguishes this saccular aneurysm from a pseudoaneurysm

aortic wall. A pseudoaneurysm (Figs. 6.2 and 6.3) or a false aneurysm is a collection of blood and connective tissue outside the aortic wall, usually the result of a rupture. A pseudoaneurysm is contained only by the periaortic tissue and not by the aortic wall itself. As previously mentioned, a pseudoaneurysm may be differentiated from a saccular aneurysm by its acute angles with the aorta or by its associated history (psuedoaneuryms are often associated with trauma).

Thoraco-abdominal aneurysms are further divided according to the Crawford classification (Fig. 6.11).[43] This classification depends on the proximal and distal extent of the aneurysm and is important for treatment decisions and for the risk--benefit analysis of various treatment options. Crawford types I and II begin at the left subclavian artery.

Crawford Classification
of
Thoraco-Abdominal Aneurysms

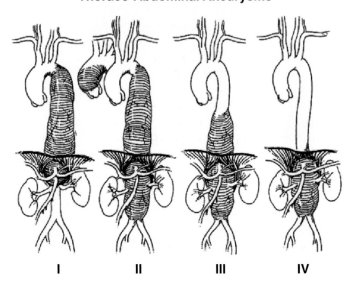

Fig. 6.11 The Crawford classification of thoraco-abdominal aortic aneurysms. See text for details. (Reproduced with kind permission from Elsevier. Copyright 2001. Society of thoracic surgeons. *Ann Thorac Surg.* 2001;71:1233–1238)

Type I extends to the renal arteries and type II extends to the aortic bifurcation. Crawford types III and IV extend to the aortic bifurcation, but type III begins in the mid thorax. Type IV begins at the diaphragm.

Although natural history data are not widely available, it has been suggested that patients with untreated large thoracic aneurysms are more likely to die of complications associated with their aneurysms than from any other cause.[44] The most important determinant of rupture is the size of the aneurysm.[45–47] Thoracic aortic aneurysms have been reported to expand at variable rates [48–50]. The American Heart Association scientific report on the surgical management of descending thoracic aortic disease reports a growth rate of 0.07 cm per year for aneurysms in the ascending aorta and aortic arch and 0.19 cm per year for aneurysm in the descending thoracic aorta.[51] If dissection complicates an aneurysm, its growth rate excels to 0.28 cm per year.[51]

The growth rate of thoracic aortic aneurysm is directly related to aneurysm size, smoking, uncontrolled hypertension, and advancing age.[51]

The anatomic location of the aneurysm is also associated with the rate of expansion. In a series of 87 patients who underwent serial computed tomography (CT) or magnetic resonance imaging (MRI), aneurysms located within the mid portion of the descending aorta showed the most rapid growth, while those in the ascending aorta had the slowest expansion rate, despite having the greatest initial diameter. The presence of thrombus, but not calcification or dissection, was also associated with accelerated growth.[48]

Asymptomatic aneurysms are initially managed medically, while surgery is indicated for those that are symptomatic, are asymptomatic but rapidly expanding, or are over 5–6 cm in diameter.

The likelihood of rupture or dissection is directly related to aneurysm size. In a prospective study of 721 patients, rupture rates varied from 2% to 7% per year for aneurysms less than 5 versus 6 cm, respectively.[49] Among patients with aneurysms 6 cm in size, the combined end point of rupture, dissection, or death occurred at a rate of 15.6% per year.[49] The 5-year rate of survival was 56% in patients with aneurysms 6 cm in size who did not undergo surgery.[50] In comparison, elective surgery restored survival to a rate similar to a matched control population.[50] Aneurysms appear to rupture at somewhat smaller sizes in patients with Marfan's syndrome.

Serial imaging of the aneurysm to evaluate growth and structural changes is recommended. The preferred imaging technique is CT angiography or magnetic resonance angiography (MRA). Imaging should be repeated at 6 months after the initial study. Further imaging can be performed at yearly intervals if there is no growth or at 3–6 months (according to aneurysm size) if there is a significant size increase from one study to another.

The indications for surgery include the presence of symptoms, asymptomatic patients with a diameter of 5–6 cm for an ascending aortic aneurysm and 6–7 cm for a descending aortic aneurysm,[52,53] accelerated growth rate (1 cm per year) in aneurysms less than 5 cm in diameter and evidence of dissection.[54]

In patients with aortic regurgitation of any severity and primary disease of the aortic root or ascending aorta (such as Marfan's syndrome), the 2006 ACC/AHA valvular disease guidelines recommend aortic valve replacement and aortic root reconstruction at a size of 5 cm.[55] The guidelines note that some have recommended surgery for this group at a lesser degree of dilatation (4.5 cm) or based on a rate of increase of 0.5 cm per year or greater in surgical centers with established expertise in repair of the aortic root and ascending aorta.[56, 57]

The 2006 ACC/AHA guidelines recommend surgery to repair the aortic root or replace the ascending aorta in patients with bicuspid aortic valves if the diameter of the aortic root or ascending aorta is greater than 5 cm or if the rate of increase in diameter is 0.5 cm per year or more. The surgical threshold in smaller patients is 5 cm.[55]

The American Heart Association recommends repair of ascending thoracic aortic aneurysms when they reach 5.5 cm and descending aortic aneurysm when they reach 6.5 cm. [349] In patients with Marfan syndrome or other genetic predisposition syndromes, consideration for repair should be given when an ascending aortic aneurysms reaches 5 cm and a descending aortic aneurysm reaches 6 cm. [349].

Figure 6.12 illustrates the typical appearance of a surgically repaired thoracic aorta.

The role of catheter-based intraluminal stent grafting in thoracic aortic disease is undergoing active clinical investigation in both elective and emergency settings. Studies to date are small and nonrandomized. The data suggest lower periprocedural complications than surgery, but higher rates of medium-term complications.

6.2.3 Surgical Management Versus Endovascular Stent Grafting

At present, intraluminal stent grafts for thoracic aneurysms are mainly available in conjunction with clinical research protocols (Figs. 6.13–6.15). In contrast, endovascular stent

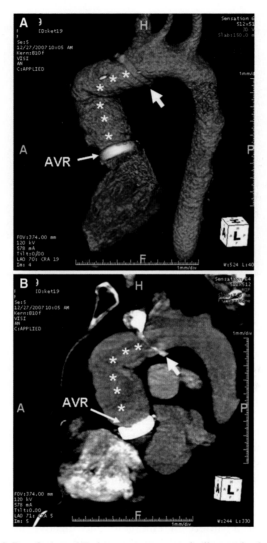

Fig. 6.12 Panels A and B demonstrate a surgically repaired ascending aorta in segmented, three-dimensional reconstruction (Panel A) and in maximum intensity projection (Panel B). The length of the graft is depicted by the *asterisks*. The aortic valve replacement (AVR) is displaced superior to the native valve annulus. The distal anastomotic ring is marked by the *thick white arrow*. Note the linear nature and sharp angles of the graft which does not look like a native aorta. This appearance is typical

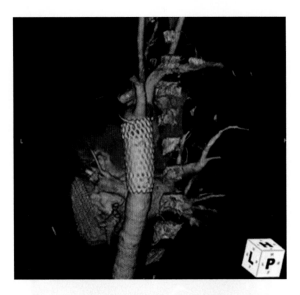

Fig. 6.13 A three-dimensional depiction of an upper descending thoracic aorta stent graft. This is the typical appearance of AneuRx stent graft

grafts are in wide and growing clinical use for the treatment of abdominal aortic aneurysms.[58–65] Figure 6.16 demonstrates an ascending endovascular stent graft with an endoleak.

Data regarding the appropriate managment of thoracic aortic disease (open surgery versus endovascular stenting) is scant and frought with limitations. A discussion of some of these data follows.

The largest published series of endovascular stenting of thoracic aortic aneurysms[63] has reported a 1-year follow-up. This study included 443 patients treated with endovascular stents for a variety of emergent and elective indications including thoracic aortic aneurysm (249 patients), thoracic aortic dissection (131 patients), traumatic aortic injury (50 patients), and false anastomotic aneurysm (13 patients). Approximately, one-third of the procedures were emergent, and one-half of the patients were deemed high risk and would not have been considered candidates for surgical repair.

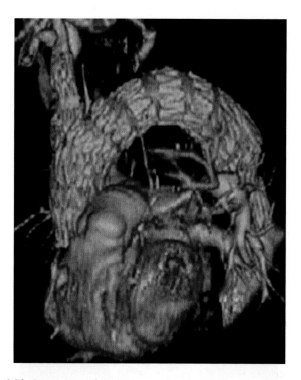

Fig. 6.14 A segmented, volume-rendered, complex thoracic aortic stent graft involving the upper ascending thoracic aorta, the entire aortic arch, and upper descending thoracic aorta. It also depicts an extension into the right brachiocephalic artery. This is the typical appearance of a Gore Excluder stent. The computed tomographic appearance of a Gore Excluder stent is similar to that of a Cook Zenith stent but the "zig zags" are smaller. (Reproduced with kind permission from HMP Communications LLC. Copyright 2000. Halawa M, Patterson B, Holt P, et al. Comparisons between thoracic stent grafts – how do we know which stent graft to select? *Vasc Dis Manag.* 2009;6[7])

Reported findings include a technical success of 87% in patients with aortic aneurysm and 89% in patients with aortic dissection. Postprocedure paraplegia occurred in 4% of aortic aneurysm patients, and in 0.8% of those with aortic dissection. Thirty-day mortality was 9.3% for the entire cohort. For

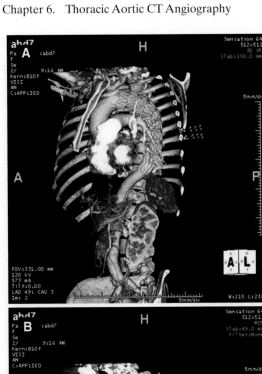

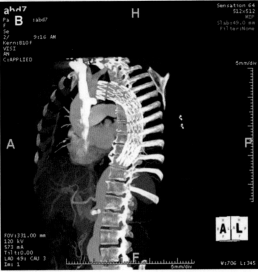

Fig. 6.15 Panel A depicts a volume-rendered image of a thoracic aortic stent beginning just after the great arch vessels and extending distally to the proximal descending thoracic aorta. This is another example of a Gore Excluder stent. Panel B is maximum intensity projection of panel A

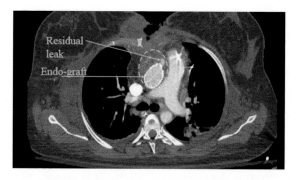

Fig. 6.16 Depiction of an endovascular ascending aortic stent graft with an endoleak. The *dotted yellow* oval represents the initial outline of the aneurysmal aorta

patients with aortic aneurysm, 30-day mortality for elective and emergent procedures was 5.3% and 28%, respectively. In those with aortic dissection, 30-day mortality for elective and emergent procedures was 6.5% and 12%, respectively. One-year mortality among patients treated for aortic aneurysm and aortic dissection was 20% and 10%, respectively.

These results are promising, but cannot be compared directly to historical outcomes following surgical repair since patients included in this series had a greater burden of comorbid disease and the short duration of follow-up precludes direct comparison with the durable effects of successful surgical repair.

The largest of the early series for which there is now medium-term follow-up was a prospective, uncontrolled study of a first-generation, custom-fabricated, self-expanding stent graft. It included 103 patients with descending thoracic aortic aneurysms, 60% of whom were not candidates for conventional surgery. Complete thrombosis of the aneurysm was achieved in 83%. Early mortality was 9% and serious complications included paraplegia in 3% and stroke in 7%. At 1.8 years of follow-up, late stent graft complications occurred in 38% and included stent graft misdeployment or removal, endoleak, aortic dissection, distal embolization, mesenteric ischemia and infection. Fatal complications occurred in 4% and included rupture of the treated aneurysm, stent graft erosion into the esophagus, arterial injury and excessive bleeding.[60]

In a subsequent report at 4.5 years of follow-up, actuarial survival at 1, 5, and 8 years were 82%, 49%, and 27%, respectively.[66] Patients who had been identified as suitable surgical candidates at the time of stent graft placement had significantly better survival at 1 year (93% versus 74%) and 5 years (78% versus 31%).[66]

In another series of 99 patients treated at a single center over a 6-year span, the overall efficacy and safety of endografts were similar to the data reported above.[65] However, outcomes improved with second-generation endografts, including a significant reduction in endoleaks (15% versus 46% with first-generation grafts), and a trend toward a lower rate of periprocedural complications (23% versus 42%) was identified.[65]

The feasibility of stenting depends on the presence of greater than 1.5 to 2 cm of normal aorta proximal and distal to the aneurysm. These areas serve as a landing zone for the stent. Straighter segments of the aorta are more successfully stented than those that are angulated. An aortic arch curvature angle of greater than 60° leads to less successful stenting of the aortic arch. In addition, adequate femoral and iliac access diameter and characteristics are mandatory. The sheath size is 20–24 French and thus the access site needs to be greater than 7 mm in diameter. Generally, the stents are oversized by 10–20%. Aggressive oversizing is not advised since folding of the stent or stent occlusion may occur. A centerline measurement is made to appropriately judge the necessary stent length. In many instances, multiple stents are required. Certain stent types may cover the great vessels of the arch.

Regarding surgical treatment, morbidity, and mortality in thoracic aortic aneurysm repair are higher than most elective surgical procedures given the anatomic constraints and operative complexity. Aortic arch aneurysm and Crawford type II aneurysms have the highest morbidity and mortality rates. Frequently, overall 30-day mortality rates exceed 10% and stroke rates are near 20% with ascending and arch aneurysm repair. Spinal and renal injury rates of 15% are reported with repair of a descending thoracic aortic aneurysm.[67, 68]

With improved technology and increased use of end-organ protection adjuncts, morbidity and mortality have decreased significantly in more recent series.[67, 69–71] Factors associated with an adverse 30-day outcome (death, paraplegia, paraparesis, stroke, or acute renal failure requiring dialysis) after thoraco-abdominal aneurysm surgery include preoperative renal insufficiency, increasing age, symptoms, and Crawford type II aneurysms.[72]

Figures 6.17 and 6.18 illustrate the Bental procedure and the Bental procedure with the Cabral modification. Both of these procedures are used to treat ascending aortic aneurysms. The Bental procedure entails replacement of the aortic root and the aortic valve with a composite graft and reimplanting the native coronary arteries onto the graft. The Cabral modification utilizes a saphenous vein graft implanted to the aortic graft with the native coronary arteries attached to the graft itself. This is particularly useful when the native coronary arteries will not reach the aortic graft.

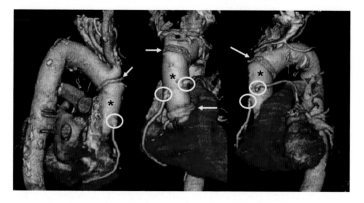

Fig. 6.17 Illustration of a segmented, volume-rendered reconstruction of a Bental procedure in multiple projection angles. The *black asterisks* depict the aortic composite graft. The *white arrows* show the suture lines of the graft. The *white circles* outline the reimplanted coronary artery to composite graft anastomoses. (Picture courtesy of Peter Fail MD. Dr. Fail is the CT medical director for Cardiology Institute of the South (CIS), Houma, Louisiana, and serves as the medical director of interventional trials for the CIS Clinical Research Corporation)

Emergency surgery for ruptured or dissected thoraco-abdominal aneurysms that have ruptured is associated with substantial morbidity and mortality. The 30-day mortality rate may approach 42%. In those that survive, postoperative complications may include renal failure (36%), respiratory failure (36%), and paraplegia or paraparesis (27‰).[73] Reoperation may be required in up to 6.6% of patients.[74] Reasons for reoperation include insufficiency or stenosis of an aortic valve replacement, true or false aneurysm formation, acute dissection, or prosthetic valve endocarditis.[74] Predictors of death after reoperation were preoperative NYHA functional class III or IV, an interval of less than 6 months between the first and second surgeries, elevated preoperative creatinine level and need for postoperative dialysis, and acute aortic dissection as indication for repeat surgery. Freedom from repetitive reoperation was 98% at 5 and 10 years.[74]

The American Heart Association scientific statement of the surgical management of descending thoracic aortic disease summarizes the data regarding open surgery versus endovascular treatment. While surgery often provides long lasting results, the traditional periperative mortality rates

Fig. 6.18 Depiction of a segmented, volume-rendered image of a Bental procedure with Cabral modification. Here, the left anterior descending (E) and the circumflex (D) coronary arteries are connected to a saphenous vein graft (B), which has been implanted onto the aortic graft. In this case, the right coronary artery (A) was reimplanted onto the aortic graft. In panel B, the saphenous vein graft is shown wrapping posteriorly around the aorta. F demonstrates the anastomotic points for the left anterior descending and circumflex onto the saphenous vein graft. C depicts the prosthetic aortic valve, which due to complicated anatomy is displaced cephalad into the aortic root. The *white line* in panel A spans the length of the aortic composite graft

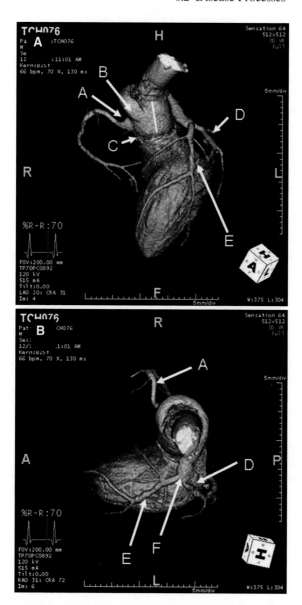

were in the 12–44% range.[51] More recent literature reflecting surgical advances reports a 4–9% periperative mortality rate with a 3% paraplegia rate for descending thoracic operations at high volume centers.[51] Advancing age correlates with a worse surgical outcome.[51]

The long-term durability of stent grafts is not optimally defined. Most studies have been limited to 5 year follow-up. In addition, stent grafts have generally been designed to last up to 10 years.[51] This durability question is not an issue for the elderly or for those that are poor surgical candidates, but becomes a big consideration in the younger patient who is otherwise a surgical candidate.

A summary of the limited comparison data available is presented in this American Heart Association scientific statement. Early studies indicate that with first generation stents, the reintervention rate by 8 years is approximately 30%.[51] However, these early data report a perioperative death rate of 2.1% versus 11.7%, respectively, with stenting versus surgery.[51] The overall stroke rate appears at this time to be similar.[51] Endoleaks occur in nearly 10% of patients.[51] Overall survival has not differed in up to 2 years of follow-up.[51]

At this time, strokes are reported to occur in 7% of endo-vascular stenting procedures with older devices and in 5.8% with newer devices.[51] Strokes are predominanty embolic and related to the atherosclerotic burden and type. Risk factors include prior stroke, advanced atherosclerosis of the aortic arch and stent graft landing zone in the distal aortic arch or the proximal descending thoracic aorta.[51] Atheroma more vulnerable to embolism are those that protrude greater than 5 mm into the aortic lumen and those that are ulcerated or pedunculated.[51] Newer devices that require less manipulation in the aortic arch cause less embolism. Appropriate patient selection and the use of newer stent devices may limit stroke.

It should be noted that thoracic aortic disease is often more diffuse than that in the abdominal aorta. Thus it may be expected that advancing disease in untreated regions may require later therapy and that further dilations at stent aposition sites may lead to future endoleaks in previously well apposed segments.

Patients with Marfan syndrome, connective tissue disease-related aneurysms, or genetic syndromes that predispose to aneurysm should not undergo endovascular treatment.[51] The aneurysm sac in patients with these syndromes has been shown to continue to expand despite exclusion with a stent due to the underlying disease process. Thus, these patients remain at risk for further complications.

At this time, the decision process regarding surgical versus endovascular treatment for thoracic aortic disease must take into account the surgical risk of the patient versus the risk of medical therapy alone and relate this to the feasibility and limitations of endovascular stenting. This decision tree must account for the patient's age.

Open surgery remains the gold standard treatment for thoracic aorta disease.[51] Until more data are available, it is not recommended to offer stent grafting to younger patients who are good surgical candidates. If endovascular therapy is considered, emphasis on patients with favorable anatomic targets is a must. The procedural risk should be lower than the surgical risk or the risk of medical therapy alone.

6.2.4 Acute Aortic Syndromes

Acute aortic syndromes are clinical emergencies caused by many factors including penetrating atherosclerotic ulcer, intramural hematoma, periaortic hematoma, aortic dissection, and aortic aneurysm.

6.2.4.1 Penetrating Atherosclerotic Ulcer

A penetrating atherosclerotic ulcer (PAU) (Figs. 6.4 and 6.19) is defined as an ulceration of an atherosclerotic aortic plaque that has penetrated through the aortic intima into the media. By definition, there is a disruption of the internal elastic lamina. Localized and variable aortic wall hematomas result. It is characterized by small, focal, contrast-filled luminal out pouchings and may be accompanied by aortic wall thickening,

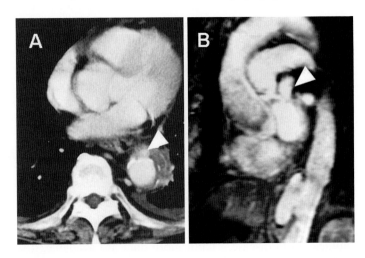

Fig. 6.19 Panels A and B illustrate maximum intensity projections penetrating aortic ulcers from two separate patients (*white arrow heads*) Note that a penetrating ulcer is contained within the atherosclerotic plaque (best seen in panel A) and remains contained within the adventitia. A psuedoaneurysm protrudes outside the aortic wall. (Reproduced with kind permission of the Radiological Society of North America. Copyright 2000. Hayashi H, Matuoka Y, Sakamoto S, et al. Penetrating atherosclerotic ulcer of the aorta: imaging features and disease concept. *Radiographics*. 2000;20:995–1005)

focal mural hematoma, and enhancement. Penetrating ulcers may progress to intramural hematoma, dissection, pseudoaneurysm, saccular aneurysm, or rupture.

Ucleration of this advanced atherosclerosis may be asymptomatic or may present like acute dissection. There is no intimal flap or extension of this process beyond the local disruption due to the advanced nature of the atherosclerosis and adjoining calcium. This may be considered a localized, focal dissection without extension.

PAU occurs far less commonly than aortic dissection (approximately 9% in one report)[349] If symtomatic at presentation, symptoms mimic dissection with intense back pain. Branch vessel involvement is rare due to the focality of this process. It is predominantly a descending thoracic aortic disease occuring in this location in nearly 90% of all cases.[349] It is also a disease of the elderly, occuring almost entirely in patients older than 65 years who have many comorbidities.[349]

The incidence of rupture is reported to be extremely high (42%) while rupture in intramural hematoma (IMH), type A dissection and type B dissection occur in 35%, 7.5% and 4.1% respectively.[349]

The appropriate treatment strategy for PAH is controversial. Data suggest that the natural history of PAH is ominous yet small trials of medical managment have yielded reasonable results.[349] Long term surgical outcomes are limited by the diffuse nature of the atherosclerotic process within the aorta. That is, areas of untreated aorta continue to progress and lead to complications.

Endovascular stenting strategies have not been well studied to date.

Since medical and surgical treatment strategies share similar long term outcomes[349] it is reasonable to treat PAH patients conservatively to start.[349] Serial imaging is necessary and should be performed within 3 to 5 days.[349] If signs of a severe bulging hematoma, extensive subadventitial spread or hematoma, increasing bloody pleural effusion or a more deeply penetrating ulcer is seen, a corrective procedure should be entertained. In addition, if any enlargement of the aorta or increased volume of hemorrhage is seen, a corrective procedure should be considered.[349]

Patients who continue to do well with a conservative strategy can continue to be surveilled using general size criteria for elective intervention.[349] If symptoms ensue, correction should be entertained.

The technical success rates and short term complication rates are favorable with endovascular stenting but no long term prognostic data or randomized prospective trials exist. Endoleaks are reported to occur in 17% of cases.[349] When choosing a treatment approach, clinical judgement and individualization of patient comorbidities and aortic characteristics should be considered. Age, long term prognosis and surgical risk are important considerations. No clear recommendations are published.

6.2.4.2 Intramural Hematoma

Intramural hematoma (IMH) is a variant of aortic dissection that is characterized by hemorrhage within the aortic media in the absence of a visible intimal tear and accounts for 5–13% of patients who present with symptoms consistent with an aortic dissection. It is generally believed that this pathology results from rupture of the vasovasorum resulting in a blood-containing space within the aortic wall with no intimal disruption. IMH is characterized by an aortic wall thickness on CT scanning of > 7 mm.[51] It does not demonstrate contrast enhancement. Less commonly it develops from a penetrating atherosclerotic ulcer or from trauma. Rarely it occurs as a result of a plaque rupture resulting in bleeding and thrombus within the media.

Intramural hematomas are more focal than aortic dissections and as a result, rarely involve branch vessels. They are more common in the descending aorta (approximately 70% of all cases)[51] and are more frequently found in the elderly.[51]

The clinical presentation is usually severe back pain. Since intramural hematomas are generally found more superficially (nearer to the adventitia), rupture is more common than in aortic dissection and occurs in up to 35% of the cases.[51] One year survival has been reported to be only 65.8%.[51] Since IMH may also progress to frank dissection and rupture, the management parallels that of a dissection.

On a CT scan without contrast, the diagnosis is made by visualizing the classic appearance of a crescent-shaped hyperattenuated region (Fig. 6.20). Displaced intimal calcification may also be seen and the aortic wall may be thickened. On a contrasted scan, a crescent-shaped or concentric hypoattenuated region is seen. Again, they do not demonstrate frank contrast enhancement with contrast injection. (Fig. 6.21).

Patients with uncomplicated IMH are generally treated like patients with uncomplicated aortic dissecton in the same aortic location. Patients with type A IMH should undergo surgery promptly and those with type B IMH may undergo an initial medical approach.

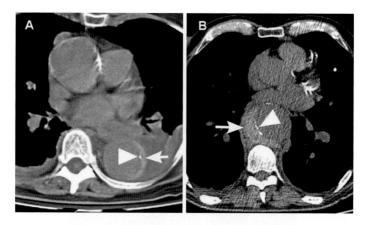

Fig. 6.20 Demonstration of intramural hematomas from two different patients seen on unenhanced scans. Panel A illustrates a crescent-shaped hyperattenuation (*white arrow*) within the arterial wall with an intimal calcification (*white arrow head*). Panel B depicts an eccentric crescent-shaped mural hyperattenuation (*white arrow*). Again, note the intimal calcifications (*arrow head*). (Reproduced with kind permission from Elsevier. Copyright 2007. Abbara S, Kalva S, Cury RC, et al. Thoracic aortic disease: spectrum of multidetector computed tomography imaging findings. *J Cardiovasc Comput Tomogr.* 2007;1(1):43–54)

Since these lesions are more fragile and prone to rupture, a low threshold of crossing from a medical to a surgical approach should be maintained. If the IMH demonstrates severe bulging, extensive subadventitial spread, extra-aortic blood, and bloody pleural effusion, then a corrective procedure should be immediately entertained.

Repeat imaging should be performed in 3–5 days.[51] If any complication noted above occurs or if there is persistent pain or an aortic size >5.5 cm, then an invasive approach is indicated. Similarly, if symptoms are not controlled with a medical approach, invasive correction should be entertained.

No randomized, controlled studies currently exist to guide the decision between surgery and endovascular stenting. Small series suggest that the technical success of an endovascular approach is high with a relatively low mortality and

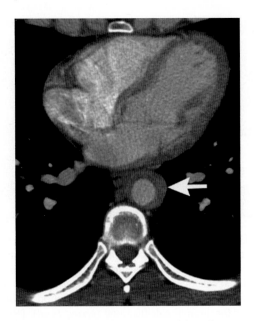

Fig. 6.21 Illustration of a contrasted scan with an intramural hematoma depicted by the *white arrow*. Note a concentric low attenuation ring around the contrasted aortic lumen

complication rate.[51] The decision on which procedure to entertain should depend on risk-benefit ratio of each procedure type individualized to the patient. This decision should take into account the aortic anatomy and the patient's age and comorbid conditions.

6.2.4.3 Periaortic Hematoma

Periaortic hematoma (Fig. 6.22), which may be detected by computed tomographic imaging, may reflect slow oozing at or near the site of an acute aortic dissection or area of blunt trauma to the aorta. It is thought to be a harbinger of impending rupture.[75]

  Periaortic hematoma occurs in up to 23% of patients presenting with signs and symptoms of aortic dissection.[75]

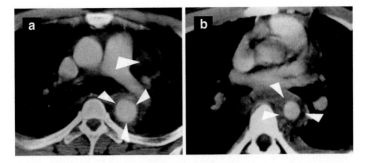

Fig. 6.22 Illustration of multiplanar reformatted, axial images of a periaortic hematoma (*arrow heads*) in two separate patients suffering blunt trauma. Panels a and b are multiplanar reformatted images. (Reproduced with kind permission from the American Roentgen Ray Society. Copyright 1998. Wong YC, Wang LJ, Lim KE, et al. Periaortic hematoma on helical CT of the chest: a criterion for predicting blunt traumatic aortic rupture. *Am J Roentgenol.* 1998;170:1523–1525)

These patients have higher rates of shock, cardiac tamponade, and altered consciousness and coma.[75] They also have a significantly higher mortality rate compared to those without a periaortic hematoma (33% versus 20%).[75] Periaortic hematomas should be treated in a similar fashion to aortic dissections located in a similar location in the aorta.

6.2.4.4 Thoracic Aortic Dissection

Aortic dissection is defined as a disruption of the media layer of the aorta with bleeding through the disruption into the aortic wall. The dissection plane is usually not more than two-thirds through the media.[51] Dissection can occur without an aneurysm vice versa. The term dissecting aortic aneurysm applies only if a dissection occurs within an aortic aneurysm. Aortic dissection is a relatively uncommon but potentially catastrophic.

Reports on the global incidence of aortic dissection vary. The American Heart Association reports an incidence of between 5 and 30 cases per million people annually,[51] which is much more frequent than abdominal aortic aneurysm rupture. Ascending aortic dissections are almost twice as common as descending dissections and the right lateral wall of the ascending aorta is the most common site of origin.[80] Aortic arch involvement is seen in up to 30%.[80] The most common patient types presenting with acute aortic dissection are 60- to 80-year-old men.[80–82] Men are effected with aortic dissection more frequently (65%) than women,[83] whose presentation tends to occur at older ages than their male counterpart.[84]

Aortic dissection is defined as a tear of the intima with free-flowing or thrombosed blood in the false lumen within the media. A false lumen is created as blood passes through the tear separating the intima from the surrounding media and adventitia. The false and true lumens are separated by an intimal flap.

Propagation of the dissection can occur both distal and proximal to the initial tear and may involve branch vessels and the aortic valve itself. The dissection may also enter the pericardial space. Such propagation is responsible for many of the associated clinical manifestations including ischemia (coronary, cerebral, spinal, or visceral), aortic regurgitation, cardiac tamponade, hemothorax, exsanguination, and death. In addition, multiple communications may form between the true and false lumen.

It is uncertain whether the initiating event in an aortic dissection is a primary rupture of the intima with secondary dissection of the media, or hemorrhage within the media and subsequent rupture of the overlying intima. Degeneration of the aortic media, or cystic medial necrosis, is felt to be a prerequisite for the development of nontraumatic aortic dissection.[80]

Intimal tear without hematoma is an uncommon variant of aortic dissection that is characterized by a linear intimal tear associated with exposure of the underlying aortic media or adventitial layers. There is no progression or separation of the medial layers.[84] Currently available imaging techniques may be unable to diagnose this type of aortic dissection because of its limited extent and because only a minimal amount of blood enters the dissected wall. However, these undetectable aortic dissections can lead to pseudoaneurysms and to aortic rupture. A high clinical index of suspicion is necessary to accurately identify this presentation type.

Predisposing factors for acute aortic dissection include advancing age, atherosclerosis, aortic aneurysm, bicuspid aortic valve, aortic coarctation, chronic hypertension, cardiovascular surgery, inflammatory disorders such as vasculitis (giant cell arteritis, Takayasu arteritis, rheumatoid arthritis, syphilitic aortitis), and collagen vascular disorders such as Marfan's syndrome, Ehlers–Danlos syndrome, and annuloaortic ectasia.[80] In addition, reports estimate that as many as 19% of patients with a thoracic aortic aneurysm and dissection have a positive family history.[80] A number of genetic mutations have been identified and are discussed in Section 6.2.2.[80]

The predisposition to aortic dissection in those with bicuspid aortic valve may relate to a congenital defect in the aortic wall resulting in the severe loss of elastic fibers in the aortic media. This leads to the aortic root and ascending aortic enlargement often associated with bicuspid aortic valves.[86–88]

Aortic coarctation may predispose to aortic dissection as well when corrective surgery leaves behind an abnormal pericoarctation aorta that has intrinsic medial faults or when balloon dilatation of native coarctation mechanically damages the inherently abnormal pericoarctation aorta. In addition, dissection may occur in the inherently abnormal aortic root above a coexisting bicuspid aortic valve. Aortic dissection or rupture, often occurring with coarctation, is an increasingly recognized cause of death in women with Turner syndrome.[89]

Rarely, aortic dissection may complicate coronary artery bypass (CABG) or heart valve replacement surgery.[90] It may occur after conventional on-pump CABG and perhaps more frequently with minimally invasive off-pump CABG (OP CABG).[91] In a review from a single institution, ascending aortic dissection occurred in 1 of 2,723 patients (0.04%) treated with conventional CABG and 3 of 308 undergoing

OP CABG (1%).[92] Cardiac catheterization with or without coronary intervention may also induce aortic dissection.[92]

Trauma rarely causes a classic dissection, but can induce a localized tear that involves all layers of the aortic wall. More commonly, chest trauma from acute deceleration (as in a motor vehicle accident or fall) results in aortic rupture.[93] The mortality rate for this type of injury is high. Less than 20% of victims reach the hospital alive.[93]

Finally, high-intensity weight lifting or other strenuous resistance training may cause acute ascending aortic dissection, possibly mediated by significant transient elevations in blood pressure.[94]

Patients with aortic dissection typically present with severe, sharp or tearing posterior chest or back pain (in dissections distal to the left subclavian) or anterior chest pain (in ascending aortic dissections). The pain can radiate anywhere in the thorax or abdomen. It can occur alone or be associated with syncope, a cerebrovascular accident, myocardial infarction, heart failure, or other clinical symptoms or signs. Hemodynamic compromise may result.

Potential neurologic manifestations include stroke or decreased consciousness due to direct extension of the dissection into the carotid arteries or diminished carotid blood flow. Alterations of consciousness are more common in women than in men.[95]

The presence of impaired or absent blood flow to peripheral vessels is manifest as a pulse deficit. These patients have a higher rate of in-hospital complications and mortality than those without a pulse deficit.[96]

Painless dissection has been reported, but is relatively uncommon.[97] A prior history of diabetes, aortic aneurysm, or cardiovascular surgery was more common in patients with painless dissection. Presenting symptoms of syncope, heart failure, or stroke were seen more often in this group. In-hospital mortality is significantly higher than for patients presenting with pain.[97] Syncope during aortic dissection is also associated with worse outcomes.[98]

Patients presenting with complaints that may be consistent with acute aortic dissection should be evaluated for pretest risk of this entity to guide diagnostic and treatment decisions.

High-risk historical features include Marfan syndrome, Loeys–Dietz syndrome, Ehlers-Danolos syndrome, Turner syndrome, other connective tissue diseases, known predisposing genetic mutations, family history of aortic dissection or aneurysm, known aortic valve disease, recent aortic manipulation such as with a catheter, and known thoracic aortic aneurysm.

High-risk clinical features are chest, back, or abdominal pain that is abrupt or instantaneous in onset, severe, and that which is described as ripping, tearing, stabbing, or sharp in quality.

High-risk physical exam features are a pulse deficit, greater than 20 mmHG difference in systolic blood pressure between one limb and another, a focal neurological deficit, and a new aortic regurgitation murmur.

Patient history and physical examination at presentation should focus on identification of these high-risk features. In patients with syncope who are at risk for aortic dissection, a focused examination for a focal neurological deficit or for pericardial tamponade should be performed. All patients presenting with neurological complaints should be assessed for the high-risk features noted above since patients presenting with neurological deficits are less likely to report chest, back, or abdominal pain.[28]

Initial evaluation should include an electrocardiogram in patients whose symptoms suggest aortic dissection. If an acute injury pattern is noted on the electrocardiogram, the patient should be treated for acute myocardial infarction without delay since this diagnosis is more common, unless the patient is at high risk for aortic dissection at which point, a dissection should first be excluded.[28]

A chest x-ray should be ordered on all intermediate and low-risk patients in order to identify alternative diagnoses that explain the symptoms or to identify findings that further raise the suspicion for an aortic dissection that may mandate further testing.[28] High-risk patients should have definitive testing which includes a transesophageal echocardiogram,

CT angiography, or magnetic resonance angiography.[28] Choice of definitive testing is based on institutional expertise and availability. In a high-risk patient where suspicion is high, a negative initial definitive test should be followed by a second definitive test.[28]

Table 6.4 depicts the initial diagnostic algorithm for patients presenting with symptoms possibly consistent with aortic dissection.[28]

TABLE 6.4 Initial diagnostic decision tree for the evaluation of a patient with symptoms that may be consistent with aortic dissection

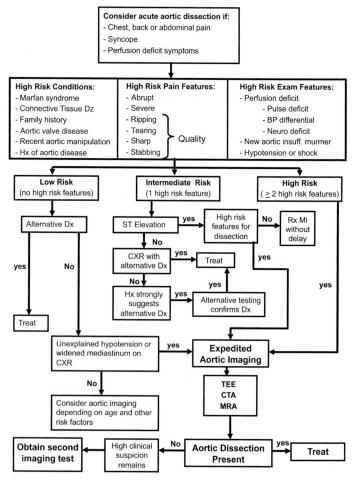

TABLE 6-5   Lists the recommended components of aortic computed tomographic (ct) imaging reporting. (27b).

1. Location of aortic abnormality

2. Maximum diameter (external wall measurement, perpendicular to the flow axis) and length of dilation.

3. For those at genetic risk for aortic disease, report measurements at the aortic valve, the sinuses of Valsalva, the sinotubular junction and the ascending aorta.

4. Comment on presence of thrombus and or atheroma

5. Comment on calcification, intramural hematoma and penetrating atherosclerotic ulcers

6. Comment on the involvement of the branch vessels and on evidence of end organ damage.

7. Note evidence of aortic rupture including periaortic and mediastinal hematoma, pericardial or pleural fluid or contrast extravasation outside the vessel lumen.

8. Direct comparison to prior imaging if available.

Table 6.5 lists the recommended components of aortic computed tomographic (CT) imaging report.[28]

Thoracic aortic dissections are characterized by two classification systems: Stanford (Daily) and Debakey systems (Table 6.6).[99–101] More widely used, the Stanford system classifies any aortic dissection involving the ascending aorta as type A, regardless of the site of the primary intimal tear. All other dissections are type B. In comparison, the Debakey system is based upon the site of origin. Type 1 originates in the ascending aorta and propagates to at least the aortic arch. Type 2 originates in, and is confined to, the ascending aorta. Type 3 originates in the descending aorta and may extend distally or proximally. Stanford Type A and Debakey types 1 and 2 are surgical emergencies because they are prone to early rupture, leading to hemopericardium, tamponade, and death. Table 6.6 also lists variant classes of aortic dissection (Fig. 6.23). Various examples of thoracic aortic dissection are illustrated in Figs. 6.24a, b, 6.25–6.31a, b (see Table 6.5).

Care must be taken not to misdiagnose a dissection when one is not present. Figure 6.32 illustrates the typical

TABLE 6.6 The Stanford, Debakey, and variant classifications of thoracic aortic dissection

Class	Description
Daily or Stanford classification	
Type A	Dissection involving the ascending aorta, regardless of primary tear site
Type B	Dissection of the descending aorta
DeBakey classification	
Type 1	Dissection of the ascending and descending thoracic aorta
Type 2	Dissection of the ascending aorta
Type 3	Dissection of the descending aorta
Classification of variants	
Class 1	Classic dissection with separation of intima/media; intimal flap between dual lumens
Class 2	Media disruption with intramural hematoma separation of intima/media; no intraluminal tear or flap
Class 3	Discrete/subtle dissection; intimal tear without hematoma (limited dissection) and eccentric bulge at tear site
Class 4	Atherosclerotic penetrating ulcer; ulcer usually penetrating to adventitia with localizing hematoma
Class 5	Iatrogenic/traumatic dissection

appearance of a pseudodissection caused by motion artifact in the ascending aorta. Note the symmetric nature of the artifact as well as a similar finding in the pulmonary artery.

Treatment options for thoracic aortic dissections have traditionally been based on these aforementioned classification systems. Surgery is usually recommended when the dissection involves the ascending aorta and medical management is preferred when the dissection involves the descending aorta,

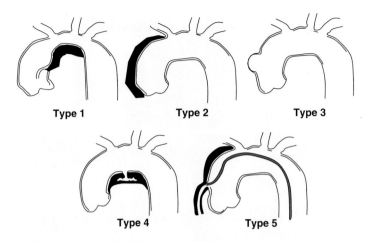

Fig. 6.23 A cartoon illustrating the five variant types of aortic dissections listed and described in Table 6.1. Type 5 illustrates trauma from engaging a coronary artery with a catheter

since operative mortality and surgical complications are more frequent with Type B dissections. Furthermore, acute complication rates with medical management alone are less common. Exceptions include malperfusion syndromes, where an invasive management approach is often necessary. Thus invasive correction for type B aortic dissections is complication driven. While surgical techniques have improved, significant morbidity and mortality may result from surgery. Furthermore, malperfusion syndromes may result from the dissection flap or from aortic rupture.[102–104] Complications occur in greater than 25% of cases after the initial surgical procedure for Type A dissections and in 60% of type B dissections.[105] The mortality rate for complications of aortic dissection approaches 50% and the morbidity rate is nearly 88%.[104]

Unfortunately, long-term outcomes with medical management alone for type B dissections are not optimal. At 5 years the mortality rate is approximately 30–50%.[51] Expansion of the false lumen occurs in 20–50% of patients at 4 years.[51] As already stated, once dissection complicates an aneurysm,

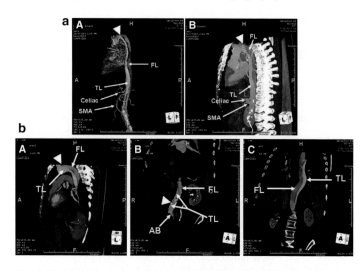

Fig. 6.24 (**a**) An example of a type III (Debakey) or Type B (Stanford) aortic dissection. The dissection begins distal to the great vessels (*white arrow head*) and extends to the distal aorta. The true lumen appears to supply the celiac artery (celiac) and the superior mesenteric artery (SMA). (**b**) Panels A, B, and C are from the same patient depicted in Fig. 6.24a. These images are maximum intensity projections. Panel A depicts the origin of the dissection flap (*white arrow head*). Panel B illustrates the end of the dissection (*white arrow head*) prior to the aortic bifurcation (AB). Panel C shows the dissection flap as it traverses the abdominal aorta. *TL* true lumen, *FL* false lumen

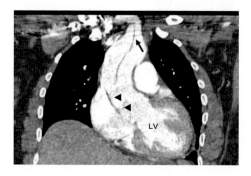

Fig. 6.25 Representation of a Debakey type II aortic dissection involving only the ascending aorta. The *black arrowheads* points to the dissection flap origins and the dissection extends into the brachio-cephalic artery (*black arrow*) but not into the aortic arch. *LV* left ventricle

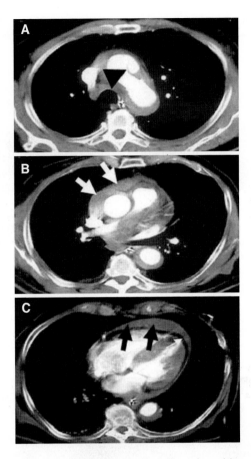

Fig. 6.26 An example of a Debakey type I dissection with rupture into the pericardium. The dissection flap is noted in panel A (*black arrow head*). The pericardial effusion is seen in panels B (*white arrows*) and C (*black arrows*). (Reproduced with kind permission from Springer Science + Business Media. Copyright 2002. Thoongsuwan N, Stern E. Chest CT scanning for clinical suspected thoracic aortic dissection: beware of the alternative diagnosis. *Emerg Radiol.* 2002;9:257–261)

growth of the aneurysm accelerates. For descending thoracic aortic dissections, expansion increases to 0.31 cm per year when there is a concomitant dissection.[51] If malperfusion syndromes such as renal failure, intestinal ischemia, or spinal ischemia occur or if contained rupture is present, urgent

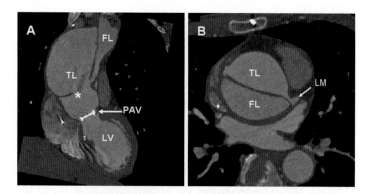

Fig. 6.27 Panels A and B show another Debakey type I dissection in multiplanar reformatted reconstructions. The dissection flap is noted by the *white asterisk* in panel A. TL represents the true lumen and FL depicts the false lumen. Panel B illustrates extension of the dissection flap into the left main coronary artery (LM). This pattern would be classified as a Beregi type 2B (Fig. 6.26). *LV* left ventricle, *PAV* prosthetic aortic valve. (Reproduced with kind permission from Elsevier. Copyright 2007. Abbara S, Kalva S, Cury R, et al. Thoracic aortic disease: spectrum of multidetector computed tomography imaging findings. *J Cardiovasc Comput Tomogr.* 2007;1:40–54)

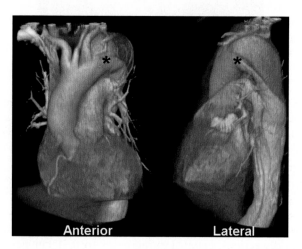

Fig. 6.28 Demonstration of a three-dimensional depiction of a Debakey type III dissection confined to the descending aorta only. The dissection flap (*black asterisks*) begins just distal to the left subclavian artery

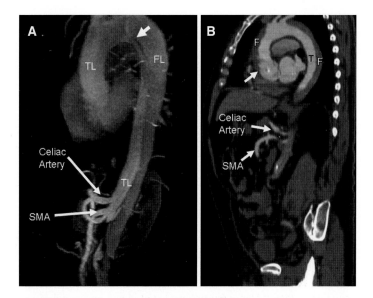

Fig. 6.29 Panel A represents a segmented, thick maximum intensity projection example of a Debakey type III dissection. The dissection flap begins (*white arrow*) at the infero-medial portion of the distal aortic arch (distal to the left subclavian). The true lumen (TL, smaller of the two lumen) perfuses the celiac artery and the superior mesenteric artery (SMA). *FL* false lumen. Panel B demonstrates a multiplanar reformatted image of a Debakey type I aortic dissection with the dissection flap beginning in the ascending aorta (*white arrow*). T represents the true lumen and F represents the false lumen. Again, the true lumen perfuses the celiac artery and the superior mesenteric artery (SMA)

repair becomes necessary, since the mortality rate rises to 20% at 2 days and to 25–50% at 1 month.[51]

Spinal ischemia occurs in 2–10% of descending aortic dissections and is not a contraindication to surgery since urgent surgery may lead to neurologic recovery.[51] While surgery is necessary for these complicated patients, surgery in these cases leads to a 14–67% risk of irreversible spinal injury or postoperative death.

Warning signs of impending rupture are recurrent pain, falling hemoglobin, rapid aortic expansion, and rapidly

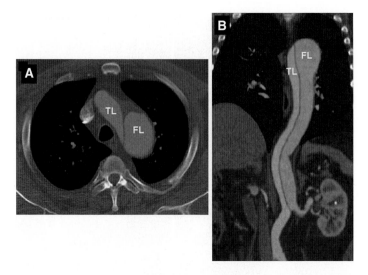

Fig. 6.30 A Debakey type III aortic dissection beginning after the aortic arch. Panel A is a multiplanar axial image and panel B is a maximum intensity coronal image. TL is the true lumen which often appears smaller. FL represents the false lumen which involves the left renal artery. (Reproduced with kind permission from Elsevier. Copyright 2007. Abbara S, Kalva S, Cury R, et al. Thoracic aortic disease: spectrum of multidetector computed tomography imaging findings. *J Cardiovasc Comput Tomogr.* 2007;1:40–54)

accumulating pleural effusion.[51] Sixty percent of deaths occur due to local rupture.[51]

The goals of invasive treatment of aortic dissection are to exclude the primary intimal tear, remove or exclude the aneurysm, and to restore and or maintain organ perfusion and major aortic side branches. While surgical and endovascular treatment options may slow the progression of disease, if any aneurysmal segment remains, the patient is at continued risk for further expansion and rupture. For this risk to be mitigated, the entire aneurysmal segments must be removed.

While surgical correction in ascending aortic dissections has been the gold standard, medical management in uncomplicated descending aortic dissection has been the most favorable treatment.

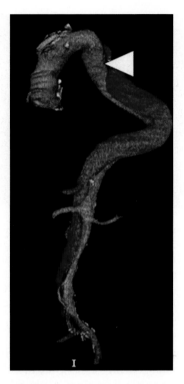

Fig. 6.31 A three-dimensional reconstruction of a Debakey type III aortic dissection. The image is a segmented, volume-rendered reconstruction. The dissection flap begins after the aortic arch in the proximal descending aorta (*white arrow head*). The true lumen is the brighter lumen. The dissection flap is seen spiraling down the aorta

Mortality rates for type B dissections treated medically have been reported to be 10.7%.[51] Surgically treated type B dissections have experienced historical mortality rates in the 31% range.[51]

Due to this outcome discrepency and since long-term outcomes with medical management alone are not optimal, endovascular approaches have become a strong consideration for the treatment of aortic dissection (as well as for aortic aneurysm as discussed previously).

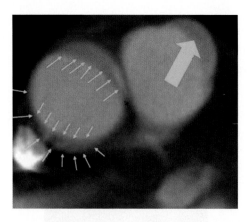

Fig. 6.32 A pseudodissection caused by motion artifact in the ascending aorta. Note the symmetric nature of the finding (*thin yellow arrows*) and the motion seen also in the pulmonary artery (*yellow block arrow*). (Picture courtesy of Peter Fail, MD. CT medical director for Cardiology Institute of the South (CIS) in Houma, Louisiana and serves as the medical director of interventional trials for the CIS Clinical Research Corporation)

However, published data guiding the choice between acute surgical management versus endovascular stenting for complicated acute aortic dissections is suboptimal. Indications for surgical correction such as refractory pain, malperfusion, rapid expansion (>1 cm per year), and maximal aneurysmal diameter of ≥5.5 cm are gaining acceptance as indications for stenting as well.

The efficacy of stenting versus surgery in the emergent setting was specifically addressed in a single-center, nonrandomized study of 60 consecutive patients with acute rupture of the thoracic aorta, where 28 patients were treated surgically and 32 were treated with an endovascular stent graft.[106] In this study, perioperative mortality was significantly lower in the stented patients (3.1% versus 17.8%). At a mean follow-up of 36 months, four additional deaths occurred in stented patients, three of which were attributed to late procedural complications (one aneurysm, one dissection, and one traumatic transection). No additional procedure-related deaths occurred in the surgical patients. Reintervention rates were similar in the two groups (three patients in each group). All of the surgical reinterventions were early reexplorations for bleeding. In the patients treated with stents, one required early drainage of an empyema and two required late interventions for endovascular leaks (one repeat stent complicated by paraplegia and one surgical repair with stent removal).

Further study in this arena is ongoing. In addition, studies evaluating the outcomes regarding prophylactic stenting in type B dissections are underway (INSTEAD trial and ADSOB trial) and should guide future therapeutic decisions.

Noninvasive imaging has led to a better understanding of the pathophysiology of ischemic complications in aortic dissection which permits more effective endovascular treatment plans and serves as a guide to optimal therapy (surgical, endovascular, or combined).[107–109] Guidance in determining the most advantageous endovascular technique to mitigate complications from dissection may be obtained by using the Beregi criteria (Fig. 6.33),[110] which attempts to identify the mechanism of the malperfusion syndrome by identifying the

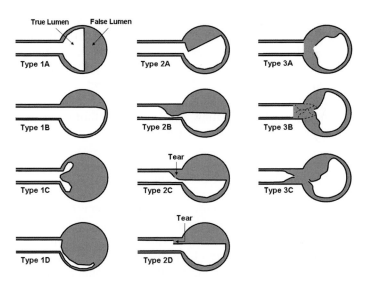

Fig. 6.33 A cartoon depicting the Beregi classification of aortic dissection. For an explanation, refer to the chapter text

intimal flap position and anatomical characteristics. The appearance of the flap as it relates to the origin of the crossing branch vessels and its extension into these branch vessels determines the optimal endovascular treatment approach.

The Beregi criteria classifies the dissection into Types I, II, and III. Each type contains its own subtypes. Type IA and Type 1C indicate flaps that are perpendicular to the branch vessel with and without compression of the true lumen, respectively. Types IB and ID represent flaps that are parallel to the branch vessel with and without compression of the true lumen. Types IIA and IIB depict a parallel flap extending into the visceral side branch with an ostial stenosis and a proximal stenosis, respectively. Type IIC represents a parallel flap extending into the side branch with a small entry tear and compression of the true lumen by increased false lumen pressure. Type IID depicts a large entry tear without compression. Type III describes an ostial evulsion with a clean tear (IIIA), persistent cobwebs (IIIB), and complete evulsion (IIIC). Many subtypes can be observed in the same patient.

Type IC or ID always require initial fenestration to equalize pressures on both sides of the flap to avoid true lumen collapse. Coexisting mechanisms often require a combination of fenestration and stenting. Most often, IIA, IIB, IIC, and IIIC mechanisms are associated with clinical or biological malperfusion and require stenting. Types IA, IB, IID, and IIIA are rarely the cause of malperfusion and thus do not require endovascular therapy.

An approach to treating and surveilling thoracic aortic disease may be viewed in tables 6.7 and 6.8.

6.2.4.5 Acute Aortic Transection

An often deadly entity, acute aortic transection is most often caused by blunt trauma such as falls or motor vehicle accidents. It results from the vertical forces on the fixed portion of the aorta relating to deceleration. The aortic injury occurs mainly at the level of the ligamentum arteriosum and proximal to the third intercostal artery (the aortic isthmus).[51]

TABLE 6.7 Lists the recommended approach to treating thoracic aortic disease.

Surgery for asymptomatic patients with ascending aortic aneurysm

Class I

1. Degenerative thoracic aneurysm, chronic dissection, intramural hematoma, penetrating atherosclerotic ulcer, mycotic aneurysm, pseudoaneurysm, otherwise healthy and have an aortic diameter of 5.5 cm or greater

2. Marfan syndrome and other genetically mediated abnormalities at diameters between 4.0 and 5.0 cm to avoid dissection or rupture

3. Patients with growth rates of more than 0.5 cm per year even if the aortic diameter is less than 5.5 cm

4. Those undergoing aortic valve replacement or repair with an aortic diameter of 4.5 cm or greater

Class IIa

1. Elective replacement for patients with Marfan syndrome, with other genetic predisposing abnormalities and with bicuspid aortic valve when the aortic root area in cm^2 divided by the patient height in meters is greater than 10

2. Elective replacement in patients with Loeys–Dietz syndrome and in patients with other TGFBR1 and TGFBR2 mutations when the aortic diameter reaches 4.2 cm or greater by internal transesophageal-measured dimensions or 4.4–4.6 cm by external CT or MRA-measured dimensions

Recommendations for aortic arch aneurysm

Class I None

Class IIa

1. Surgical repair in patients with ascending aortic aneurysm that include the proximal arch

2. Arch replacement for acute dissecton in an aneurysmal arch with extensive destruction and leakage

3. Arch replacement for aneurysms involving the entire arch, chronic dissections in an enlarged arch, distal arch aneurysm involving the descending thoracic aorta using an elephant trunk procedure

4. Arch replacement in low operative risk patients in whom the arch diameter exceeds 5.5 cm

(continued)

TABLE 6.7 (continued)

5. Reimage isolated arch aneurysms with CT or MRA in 1 year intervals if the aneurysm is less than 4.0 cm

6. Reimage isolated arch aneurysms with CT or MRA at 6 month intervals if the aneurysm is greater than or equal to 4 cm

Repair for Descending Thoracic Aorta and Thoracoabdominal Aortic Aneurysm

Class I

1. Chronic dissection especially if associated with a connective tissue disease, if good surgical risk, when the aortic diameter exceeds 5.5 cm

2. Consider endovascular stenting in patients with degenerative or traumatic aneurysm, saccular aneurysm or postoperative pseudoaneurysms when they exceed 5.5 cm

3. Consider surgery for thoracoabdominal aneurysms when endovascular options are limited and the patient is not an optimal surgical risk when the aortic diameter reaches 6.0 cm or greater

4. Additional revascularization in patients with thoracoabdominal aneurysm with end organ ischemia

TABLE 6.8 Depicts the recommended approach to thoracic aortic disease surveillance.

Class I None

Class IIa

1. CT angiography or MRA after a type A or B aortic dissection or after a repair of the aortic root or ascending aorta

2. CT angiography or MRA at 1, 3, 6, and 12 months postdissection and if stable, annually thereafter

3. Utilize the same modality at the same institution for repeated surveillance

4. MRA is recommended if possible for surveillance in medium-sized aneurysms to limit radiation exposure

5. Surveillance for intramural hematoma should be similar to that of aortic dissection

The injury results in a variety of pathologies ranging from a simple subintimal hemorrhage with or without intimal laceration to a complete transection.[51] Aortic transection usually results in death at the scene of the accident (85%).[51] Approximately 15–20% of patients make it to the hospital.[51] In the ensuing 48 h, patients die at a rate of 1% per hour in the absence of an intervention.[51] Of the patients that present to the hospital, 33% are under hemodynamic distress.[51] The overall mortality of these patients in hemodynamic distress is nearly 100%.[51] Of those that present to the hospital in stable condition, 25% will ultimately die.[51] Traumatic aortic transection is rarely an isolated problem. Most patients have a multitude of other injuries with which to contend.[51]

The pathology in those that reach the hospital is usually an incomplete noncircumferential tear limited to the intima and media.[51] The rupture is contained by the strength of the adventitia and the periaortic tissue.[51]

A 16 slice or greater CT scanner is recommended to make this diagnosis since the sensitivity of this type of scanner approaches 100%.[51] Transesophageal echocardiography is less sensitive and invasive angiography is reserved for indeterminant CT results.[51]

The standard treatment of acute aortic transection involves rapid identification and surgical correction to minimize the risk of impending rupture.[51] The operative mortality approaches 18–28%.[51] The paraplegia rate perioperatively is reported to reach up to 14%. The severe nature of the associated injuries may explain the high rate of perioperative death.

Patients with advanced age, multiple comorbidities, and a higher than normal surgical risk may be candidates for non-operative management. Some studies have demonstrated relative safety using a conservative strategy of delayed operative management.[51] However, up to 10% of these patients die while waiting for a definitive procedure.[51] Serial imaging studies are recommended to look for worsening signs of enlarging mediastinal hematoma and worsened pleural effusions which may force surgery.

Since in many patients the surgical risk outweighs the risk of a conservative approach, endovascular stenting in acute aortic transection may be an option. No randomized, prospective studies exist, but small retrospective studies have been published. These limited experiences have demonstrated stent grafting to be a safe alternative in selective cases.[51] Endoleaks do occur and the left subclavian artery often needs to be covered (>80%).[51] However, immediate periprocedural death rates and paraplegia rates are lower than with surgery in these studies.[51]

Since patients with acute aortic transection are often younger with less atherosclerosis and generally with smaller diameter aortas, smaller stents are required than when treating aneurysm or dissections.[51] In addition, smaller diameter arches may make this procedure technically more difficult.[51]

Additional study is necessary to further determine the optimal treatment strategy in these patients.

6.2.5 Aortic Coarctation

Coarctation of the aorta (Fig. 6.34) is a developmental disorder that occurs when there is partial involution of the left dorsal aortic arch. Preductal coarctation occurs when the involution occurs cranial to the left sixth branchial arch and postductal coarctation occurs when involution occurs distally.[111] Aortic coarctation is associated with bicuspid aortic valves and thoracic aortic aneurysms. Cystic medial degeneration is also implicated in thoracic aortic aneurysm associated with coarctation. Rib notching may occur due to intercostal collaterals. The treatment of choice is surgical correction with a patch closure of the coarctation which has about a 5% incidence of aneurysm formation and requires yearly CT surveillance. Endovascular stenting is also feasible (Figs. 6.35 and 6.36). Pseudocoarctation (Fig. 6.37) is a normal variant that results from a high arch with pseudokinking of the elongated aorta where it is tethered by the ligamentum arteriosum.

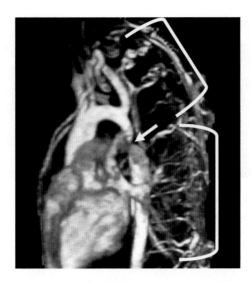

Fig. 6.34 A black and white segmented, volume-rendered depiction of a coarctation of the aorta (*white arrow*). The white brackets outline the vast collaterals that have formed to compensate

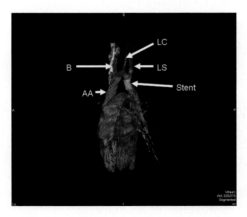

Fig. 6.35 An endovascular correction of a symptomatic coarctation of the aorta using a stent. The image is a segmented, volume-rendered reconstruction. (Image provided courtesy of Russel Hirsch, MD, Assistant Professor and Director of the Cardiac Catheterization Laboratory, Cincinnati Children's Medical Center, Cincinnati, Ohio)

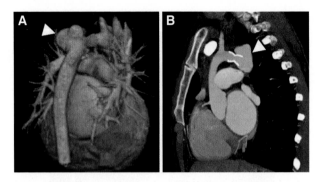

Fig. 6.36 Illustration of the late complications of a surgical coarcta-tion repair. The initial repair was performed using a left subclavian artery patch. Restenosis subsequently developed and a stent was placed with subsequent development of an aneurysm at the location of the initial patch repair, *white arrow heads* in both panels A and B. Panel A is a volume-rendered image and panel B is a maximum intensity projection. (Reproduced with kind permission from Elsevier. Copyright 2007. Abbara S, Kalva S, Cury R, et al. Thoracic aortic disease: spectrum of multidetector computed tomography imaging findings. *J Cardiovasc Comput Tomogr* 2007;1:40–54)

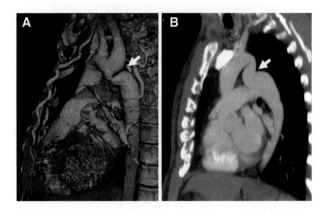

Fig. 6.37 An example of a pseudocoarctation (*white arrows*). Panel A is the volume-rendered image and panel B is the maximum inten-sity projection. (Reproduced with kind permission from Elsevier. Copyright 2007. Abbara S, Kalva S, Cury R, et al. Thoracic aortic disease: spectrum of multidetector computed tomography imaging findings. *J Cardiovasc Comput Tomogr.* 2007;1:40–54)

6.2.6 Inflammatory and Infectious Disorders

A broad grouping of inflammatory and infectious disorders, classified under aortitis, may affect the thoracic aorta. These disorders can occasionally cause aortic aneurysm as well. Giant cell arteritis, syphilitic aortitis, and mycotic aneurysm often due to bacterial endocarditis, Takayasu arteritis, rheumatoid arthritis, psoriatic arthritis, ankylosing spondylitis, reactive arthritis, and Wegener's granulomatosis are among the inflammatory and infectious disorders that affect the thoracic aorta and its branches. The common pathology in these disorders is intramural inflammation and degeneration either in response to an infectious agent or to a systemic autoimmune process. Those inflammatory diseases associated with aortic aneurysm and dissection include Giant Cell arteritis, Takayasu arteritis, Bechet disease, and Ankylosing spondylitis. Giant Cell arteritis and Takayasu arteritis are described below.

6.2.6.1 Giant Cell Arteritis

Giant cell arteritis (GCA) (Fig. 6.38) is a chronic vasculitis of large and medium-sized vessels. The mean age at diagnosis is approximately 72 years. Age is the greatest risk factor for the development of GCA.[112] The disease almost never occurs in individuals younger than 50.[112] Among individuals older than 50, the prevalence of GCA has been estimated to be 1 in 500 individuals.[113] In addition to age, female gender is a risk factor for GCA, since females are affected more frequently than males.[113]

The following classification criteria[114] is used to distinguish GCA from other forms of vasculitis: age greater than or equal to 50 years at the time of disease onset, new onset of a localized headache, tenderness or decreased pulse in the temporal artery, erythrocyte sedimentation rate (ESR) greater than 50 mm/h, and a biopsy revealing a necrotizing arteritis with a predominance of mononuclear cells or a granulomatous process with multinucleated giant cells. The presence of

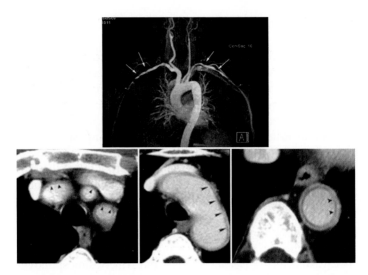

Fig. 6.38 Two examples of giant cell arteritis. The upper panel is from one patient. It depicts multiple, smooth stenoses of the large thoracic and upper extremity arteries such as the subclavian arteries (*white arrows*). The lower three panels are from a separate patient and demonstrate diffuse thickening of the arterial walls of the great vessels (*black arrow heads*) including the brachiocephalic artery, the left carotid artery and left subclavian artery (*left panel* from left to right), the aortic arch (*middle panel*), and the descending aorta (*right panel*). (Reproduced with kind permission from the American Roentgen Ray Society. Copyright 2003. Bau J, Ly J, Borstad G, et al. Giant cell arteritis. *AJR Am J Roentgenol.* 2003;181(3):742)

three of these five criteria is associated with a 94% sensitivity and a 91% specificity for the diagnosis of GCA.[114]

GCA is a systemic illness and vascular involvement may be widespread. However, blood vessel inflammation most frequently involves the arteries that originate from the aortic arch as well as the cranial arteries.[115,116] Thoracic aortic aneurysm formation occurs in up to 11% of patients with GCA and may be associated with aortic dissection which is usually a late manifestation that can occur in an otherwise asymptomatic patient.[117] As a result, yearly surveillance chest x-rays are recommended for up to 10 years to identify patients with thoracic aortic aneurysms prior to rupture or dissection. Visual loss may also result from cranial arteritis.

Symptom onset in GCA is often gradual, but abrupt presentations do occur. Systemic symptoms include fever (often low grade), fatigue, and weight loss. High-grade fevers may occur. In nearly 10% of patients, constitutional symptoms and/or laboratory evidence of inflammation are the only clues to the presence of GCA.[118,119] A new headache is common.[119] Nearly half of GCA patients experience disabling jaw claudication that occurs rapidly after beginning to chew.[119]

A variety of visual manifestations occur in GCA.[120] Ocular involvement may begin with amaurosis fugax which is caused by transient ischemia of the retina, choroid, or optic nerve. Ischemic optic neuropathy, central or branch retinal arterial occlusion, choroidal infarction, and blindness may follow.[120] Blindness occurs in 15–20% of GCA patients.[113]

Approximately, 3–15% of patients may experience arm claudication due to involvement of the subclavian and axillary arteries.[119, 121] A gradual tapering of these vessels is typical.[121, 122] Aortic aneurysms may also develop late in the disease process, resulting from chronic or late aortitis and from mechanical stress on the weakened aortic wall. Ongoing surveillance imaging is required to identify this potentially serious complication.[121] Despite this, aortic dissection can occur in the absence of aneurysmal dilation.[117]

Documented involvement of intracranial vessels in GCA is rare.[123] When transient ischemic attacks, vertigo, hearing loss, and stroke occur in GCA, they are most often due to vertebral artery or internal carotid artery involvement.[123] Carotid and vertebro-basilar involvement may also result from aortic dissection. Vertebral artery disease is more common than carotid involvement.

6.2.6.2 Takayasu Arteritis

Takayasu arteritis (Fig. 6.39) is a chronic vasculitis of unknown etiology with a worldwide distribution. However, it is most

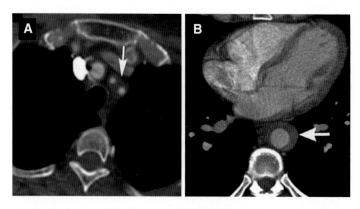

Fig. 6.39 Panels A and B represent an example of Takayasu arteritis. Panel A shows severe concentric thickening of the arterial walls of the left carotid and left subclavian arteries, *white arrow*. In addition, arterial narrowing is observed. Panel B shows similar findings in the descending thoracic aorta (*white arrow*). Clinical criteria such as patient age are often the only methods to distinguish Takayasu arteritis from giant cell arteritis as anatomically they are similar in appearance. (Reproduced with kind permission from Elsevier. Copyright 2007. Abbara S, Kalva S, Cury R, et al. Thoracic aortic disease: spectrum of multidetector computed tomography imaging findings. *J Cardiovasc Comput Tomogr.* 2007;1:40–54)

prevalent in Asia.[124] Women are affected in 80–90% of cases.[125, 126] The usual age of onset is between 10 and 40 years.[125, 126]

The primary focus of Takayasu arteritis is the aorta and its primary branches.[127] Disease expression is variable. The inflammation and arterial wall thickening may either involve the entire aorta or localize itself to a portion of the thoracic or abdominal aorta and branches.[128] The initial vascular lesions frequently occur in the left subclavian artery and often progress to the left carotid, vertebral, and brachio-cephalic arteries.[129] The right subclavian, carotid, and verte-bral arteries may also be affected.[129] The abdominal aorta and pulmonary arteries are involved in approximately 50% of patients. The proximal aorta may become dilated secondary to inflammatory injury.[129]

Narrowing, occlusion, or dilation of involved arterial segments results in a wide variety of symptoms.[129] Systemic symptoms are common in the early phase of Takayasu arteritis and may include fatigue, weight loss, and low-grade fever. Other nonvascular manifestations of Takayasu arteritis include arthralgias, myalgias, and synovitis. Skin lesions resembling erythema nodosum or pyoderma gangrenosum may occur.

Vascular symptoms are rare at presentation. As the disease progresses, however, vascular symptoms become evident and may include cold extremities and arm or leg claudication. Subclavian artery involvement is common and a stenosis proximal to the vertebral artery may lead to the subclavian steal syndrome. In advanced cases, arterial occlusion may lead to ischemic ulcerations or gangrene.

Involvement of the carotid and vertebral arteries can lead to vertigo, syncope, orthostasis, headaches, convulsions, and dementia. Visual impairment is a late manifestation. Mesenteric artery ischemia may result in abdominal pain, diarrhea, and gastrointestinal hemorrhage. Angina pectoris occurs when coronary artery ostial narrowing from aortitis or coronary arteritis is present. Myocardial infarction may occur. Pathological pulmonary artery involvement is seen in up to half of the cases. Pulmonary manifestations may include chest pain, dyspnea, hemoptysis, and pulmonary hypertension.

The American College of Rheumatology has established classification criteria for Takayasu arteritis which is designed to distinguish this disorder from other forms of vasculitis.[126] At least three of the following six criteria are necessary to diagnose Takayasu arteritis: (1) Age at disease onset of 40 years or greater. (2) Claudication of the extremities. (3) Decreased pulse in one or both brachial arteries. (4) A difference of at least 10 mmHg in systolic blood pressure between the arms. (5) A bruit over one or both subclavian arteries or the abdominal aorta. (6) Arteriographic narrowing or occlusion of the aorta, its primary branches, or of the proximal portions of the large upper and lower extremity arteries. This classification system yields a sensitivity and specificity of 90.5% and 97.8%, respectively.[126]

6.2.7 Developmental Abnormalities of the Great Vessels[130–132]

6.2.7.1 Great Arteries

Congenital abnormalities of the thoracic vascular system are common. Knowledge of their embryologic etiology may be helpful in understanding and diagnosing these anomalies.
Initially, the embryo has two dorsal aortae that communicate with an aortic sac via several pairs of branchial arch arteries which arise and involute at various times during development (Fig. 6.40). The aortic sac communicates with the heart through the truncus arteriosus which later divides into the

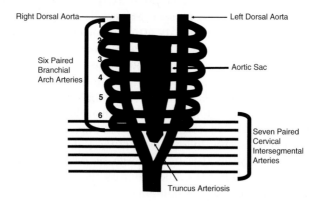

Fig. 6.40 A cartoon of the paired dorsal aortae, the six paired branchial arch arteries, the aortic sac, and the seven paired cervical intersegmental arteries that eventually transform into the aortic arch and the great vessels. See text for details

pulmonary trunk and the ascending aortas. The primitive pattern is transformed to the adult pattern by involution of particular vascular segments (Fig. 6.41a, b). Normally, the first, second, and fifth aortic arches involute.

The seven paired intersegmental arteries emanate from the dorsal aortae. The left fourth arch becomes the transverse aortic arch and the right fourth arch becomes the root of the right subclavian artery. The left sixth arch becomes the ductus arteriosus. The left subclavian arteries are derived from the seven paired intersegmental arteries arising from the aorta. The right fourth arch along with the right seventh intersegmental artery forms the right subclavian artery.

The aortic sac develops into the brachiocephalic trunk. Anterior to the third branchial arches, the dorsal aortae persist to form the common carotids. Behind the third arch, the right dorsal aorta disappears to the point where the two dorsal aortae fuse to form the descending aorta. The left dorsal aorta between the third and fourth arches disappears and the remainder forms the descending part of the aortic arch.

Aortic arch anomalies are rare and account for 1–3% of congenital heart disease and may be incidental or symptomatic.[133] Usually, symptoms result from the formation of vascular rings and slings resulting from these congenital anomalies. A vascular ring or sling results from a variety of congenital vascular abnormalities that encircle or compress the esophagus and trachea and may be complete or incomplete. Most result from abnormalities of the aortic arch and its branch arteries except the pulmonary artery sling (Fig. 6.42a, b).

Males are 1.4–2 times more likely to have vascular rings than females.[134] The clinical symptoms are most commonly respiratory and result from compression of the trachea or bronchi. Symptoms include inspiratory stridor and wheezing, dyspnea, chronic cough, and recurrent respiratory infections. Gastrointestinal symptoms may also result from esophageal compression and include dysphagia and emesis.

Most complete rings (>90%) are caused by a double aortic arch or a right aortic arch with aberrant left subclavian artery

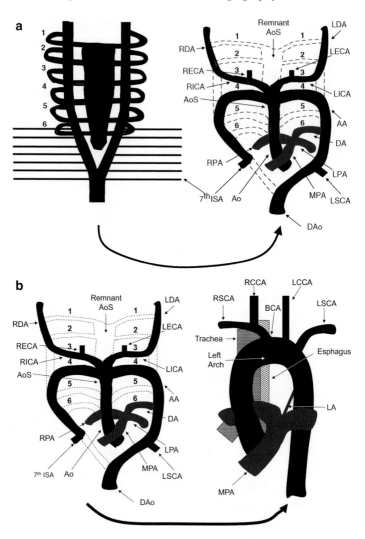

with left ligamentum arteriosum (Figs. 6.43a, b, 6.44a, b, 6.45, and 6.46).[135] These anomalies completely encircle the trachea and esophagus and may compress them. Figure 6.47 demonstrates an aberrant left common carotid artery which may cause a vascular ring as well. Figure 6.48 depicts a very

← ——————————————————

Fig. 6.41 (**a**) Illustration of the normal arch transformation by the appropriate involution of the branchial arteries and intersegmental arteries. *RDA* right dorsal aorta, *LDA* left dorsal aorta, *AoS* aortic sac, *RECA* right external carotid artery, *LECA* left external carotid artery, *RICA* right internal carotid artery, *LICA* left internal carotid artery, *AA* aortic arch, *DA* ductus arteriosus, *RPA* right pulmonary artery, *LPA* left pulmonary artery, *MPA* main pulmonary artery, *LSCA* left subclavian artery, *DAo*, descending aorta, *Ao* aorta, *ISA* intersegmental artery, Numbers 1 to 6 represent the branchial arches. *Dotted lines* represent involution of a branchial arch. *RSCA* right subclavian artery, *BCA* brachio-cephalic artery, *RCCA* right common carotid artery, *LCCA* left common carotid artery, *LSCA* left subclavian artery, *LA* ligamentum arteriosum. (**b**) Illustration of the normal arch transformation by the appropriate involution of the branchial arteries and intersegmental arteries. *RDA* right dorsal aorta, *LDA* left dorsal aorta, *AoS* aortic sac, *RECA* right external carotid artery, *LECA* left external carotid artery, *RICA* right internal carotid artery, *LICA* left internal carotid artery, *AA* aortic arch, *DA* ductus arteriosus, *RPA* right pulmonary artery, *LPA* left pulmonary artery, *MPA* main pulmonary artery, *LSCA* left subclavian artery, *DAo* descending aorta, *Ao* aorta, *ISA*, intersegmental artery, Numbers 1 to 6 represent the branchial arches. *Dotted lines* represent involution of a branchial arch. *RSCA* right subclavian artery, *BCA* brachiocephalic artery, *RCCA* right common carotid artery, *LCCA* left common carotid artery, *LSCA* left subclavian artery, *LA* ligamentum arteriosum

complex vascular anomaly which also depicts an aberrant left common carotid artery from the ascending aorta. Figure 6.49a, b demonstrates an anomalous right subclavian artery causing a vascular ring. Incomplete rings arise from an aberrant right subclavian artery, an anomalous innominate artery, a pulmonary vascular sling, and a right aortic arch with mirror image branching.

A double aortic arch results when the most caudal portion of the right dorsal aorta does not involute and the right and left branchial arches persist.[131] The right common carotid and right subclavian arteries usually arise from the rightward arch and the left common carotid and left subclavian arteries arise from the leftward arch. The ductus arteriosus may arise from

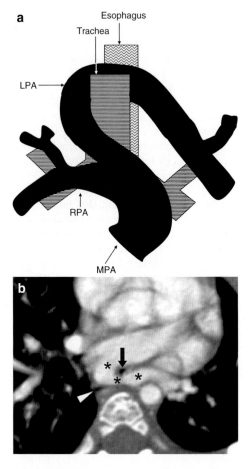

Fig. 6.42 (**a**) A cartoon demonstrating a pulmonary sling where, in this example, the left pulmonary artery wraps behind the trachea and in front of the esophagus causing tracheal compression. *LPA* left pulmonary artery, *RPA* right pulmonary artery, *MPA* main pulmonary artery. (**b**) A pulmonary sling. The left pulmonary artery (*black asterisks*) courses behind the trachea (*black arrow*) and causes compression and stridor. (Reproduced with kind permission from Radiological Society of North America. Copyright 2003. Woo Goo H, Park IS, KonKo J, et al. CT of congenital heart disease: normal anatomy and typical pathologic conditions. *Radiographics*. 2003;23:S147–S165)

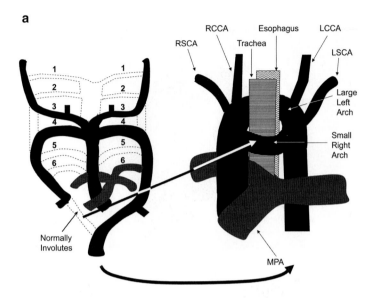

Fig. 6.43 (**a**) Demonstration of the developmental aberrations that cause a double aortic arch (failure to involute of the distal right dorsal aorta in the posterior aortic arch). The numbers 1 to 6 represent the branchial arches. *Dotted lines* represent involution. *RSCA* right subclavian artery, *LSCA* left subclavian artery, *RCCA* right common carotid artery, *LCCA* left common carotid artery. (**b**) An axial, maximum intensity projection of a double aortic arch. The *white arrows* identify the posterior arch and the *white arrow heads* point to the anterior arch. These two arches surround the trachea and esophagus. *T* trachea, *E* esophagus. (Panel b reproduced with kind permission of Elsevier. Copyright 2007. Abbara S, Kalva S, Cury R, et al. Thoracic aortic disease: spectrum of multidetector computed tomography imaging findings. *J Cardiovasc Comput Tomogr*. 2007;1:40–54)

b

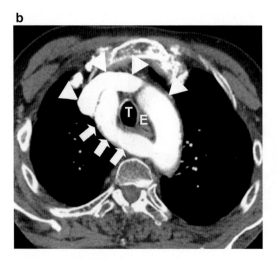

Fig. 6.43 (continued)

either arch or from both arches. A single left ductus is most often seen. Usually, the right arch is larger and more cephalad.[135] Figure 6.50 is another example of a double aortic arch.

Another interesting aortic arch anomaly is the persistent fifth branchial arch. This condition has two distinct forms.[136] The first is the systemic to systemic type, where the persistent fifth branchial arch emanates from the aortic arch at the origin of the right brachiocephalic artery and connects with the aorta more distally in the proximal descending aorta.[136] The second form is a systemic to pulmonary artery connection, where the anomalous branch reconnects with the pulmonary artery resulting in left to right shunt physiology and symptomatology.[136]

This anomaly is rare and is often associated with ventricular septal defects, pulmonic stenosis or atresia, isolated infundibuloarterial inversion, and interruption of the aortic arch or aortic coarctation.[136]

Figure 6.51 depicts a systemic to systemic example of a persistent fifth branchial arch.

A right-sided aortic arch forms when the entire right dorsal aortic arch persists and a segment of the left aortic arch

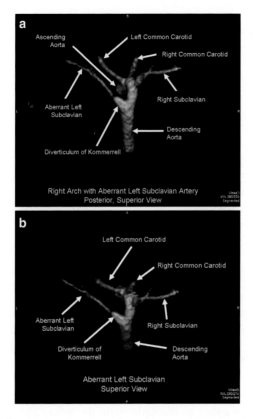

Fig. 6.44 (**a**) A posterior view of a volume-rendered depiction, segmented reconstruction of a right-sided aortic arch with an anomalous, posterior coursing left subclavian artery emanating from a diverticulum of Kommerell located on the descending aorta. This anomaly may cause a vascular ring (Image provided courtesy of Russel Hirsch, MD, Assistant Professor and Director of the Cardiac Catheterization Laboratory, Cincinnati Children's Medical Center, Cincinnati, Ohio). (**b**) A superior view of the same volume-rendered, segmented image in (**a**). (Image provided courtesy of Russel Hirsch, MD, Assistant Professor and Director of the Cardiac Catheterization Laboratory, Cincinnati Children's Medical Center, Cincinnati, Ohio)

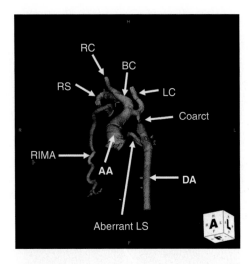

Fig. 6.45 A segmented, volume-rendered depiction of a left-sided aortic arch with an aberrant left subclavian artery (LS) emanating from the descending aorta. There is a coarctation (coarct) of the aorta noted with a concomitantly hypertrophied right internal mammary artery (RIMA). *AA* ascending aorta, *RS* right subclavian artery, *BC* brachiocephalic artery, *RC* right carotid artery, *LC* left carotid artery, *DA* descending aorta

disappears. The arch lies to the right of the spine before descending either to the right or to the left of the spine.[131] A left or right arch is defined by the main stem bronchus that is crossed by the aortic arch not by the side on which the aorta descends. Therefore, a right aortic arch crosses the right main stem bronchus and vice versa. At times, no ring or sling occurs if there is no retroesophageal component (Fig. 6.52).

Two types of right aortic arch anomalies exist. The first is the right aortic arch with mirror image branching. This anomaly may or may not cause compression of the trachea and esophagus depending on the location of the ligamentum arteriosum. In this anomaly, the arch gives rise to three branches, the right brachiocephalic trunk, the right common carotid artery, and the right subclavian artery, mirroring the left arch anatomy. The left common carotid artery and the left subclavian arise from

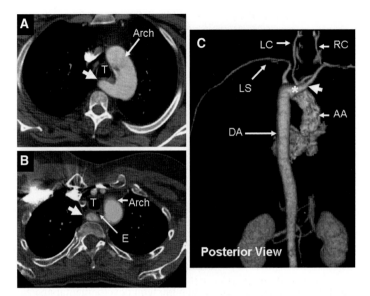

Fig. 6.46 Depiction of a left aortic arch with an anomalous right subclavian artery (*thick white arrows*) emanating distally and posteriorly from a diverticulum of Kommerell (*white asterisk* in panel C) and coursing posteriorly forming a vascular ring. Panels A and B are multiplanar reformatted images where "Arch" represents the aortic arch, "T" is the trachea, "E" is the esophagus and *thick white arrows* point to the aberrant right subclavian artery. Panel C is a volume-rendered image. The *white star* is the Diverticulum of Kommerell. (Reproduced with kind permission of Elsevier. Copyright 2007. Abbara S, Kalva S, Cury R, et al. Thoracic aortic disease: spectrum of multidetector computed tomography imaging findings. *J Cardiovasc Comput Tomogr.* 2007;1:40–54)

elsewhere on the aorta. Mirror image right arches may form both complete and incomplete vascular rings.

Figure 6.53 demonstrates a mirror image right aortic arch with both a complete and an incomplete ring.

The second type of right aortic arch is the right aortic arch with aberrant left subclavian artery and left ligamentum arteriosum. Here, a complete ring is formed by the right arch, the anomalous left subclavian artery, and the left-sided

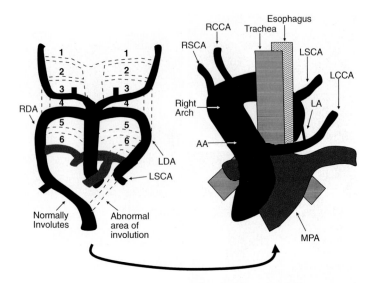

Fig. 6.47 A cartoon demonstrating the fetal developmental aberrations responsible for a right aortic arch with an anomalous left common carotid artery emanating from the ascending aorta and coursing anteriorly forming a vascular ring. This anomaly is caused by abnormal involution of the distal part of the left dorsal aorta and persistence of the distal part of the right dorsal aorta which normally involutes. Numbers 1 to 6 represent the branchial arches and the dotted lines represent involution. *RDA* right dorsal arch, *LDA* left dorsal arch, *RSCA* right subclavian artery, *RCCA* right common carotid artery, *LSCA* left subclavian artery, *LA* ligamentum arteriosum, *LCCA* left common carotid artery, *MPA* main pulmonary artery, *AA* ascending aorta

ligamentum arteriosum attached to the aberrant left subclavian artery. Figure 6.54 depicts this anomaly.

Left subclavian anomalies may often arise from a vascular structure known as Kommerell's diverticulum, which may contribute to the compression of the esophagus and trachea. Kommerell's diverticulum may be found in many different aortic arch anomalies, but is most often seen with a right aortic arch with an aberrant left subclavian artery (Fig. 6.54a, b). Kommerell's diverticulum results from regression of the fourth left aortic arch.[137]

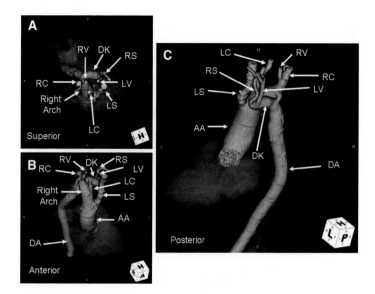

Fig. 6.48 Depiction of volume-rendered, segmental reconstructions of a right aortic arch with complex vascular anomalies, some of which are diagramed in the cartoon in Fig. 6.47. Panel A is a superior view, panel B is an anterior view, and panel C is a posterior view. In this example, the left subclavian artery (LS) is the first vessel arising from the ascending aorta. It is followed by the left carotid artery (LC). The aortic arch then travels rightward where the right vertebral artery (RV) and the right carotid artery (RC) arise. Further along the arch arises a diverticulum of Kommerell (DK) which gives rise to the left vertebral artery (LV) and the right subclavian artery (RS), which courses posteriorly to its normal position, thus forming a ring

A cervical aortic arch (Fig. 5.9) is characterized by an arch that extends cephalad into the upper mediastinum or lower cervical region. Its embryologic etiology is debated in the literature. Its branches are variable, but often, the right subclavian and the internal and external carotid arteries arise separately from the arch.[131]

Other causes of complete vascular rings include a left aortic arch with a right descending aorta and right ligamentum arteriosum, a right aortic arch with a left descending aorta and left ligamentum arteriosum, and a left aortic arch with an

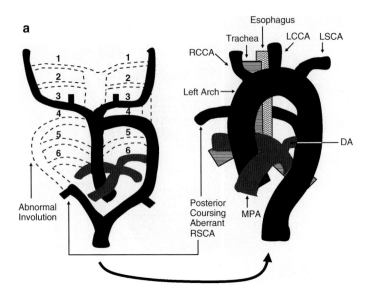

Fig. 6.49 (**a**) A cartoon of a vascular ring composed of an aberrant right subclavian artery coursing posteriorly to its normal position, thus forming a vascular ring. The left side of the cartoon depicts the aberrant fetal development that results in this anomaly. Numbers 1 to 6 represent the branchial arches. The *dotted lines* represent involution. This anomaly results from abnormal involution of part of the right dorsal aorta. *RSCA* right subclavian artery, *RCCA* right common carotid artery, *LCCA* left common carotid artery, *LSCA* left subclavian artery, *DA* ductus arteriosus, *AA* ascending aorta, *Desc Ao* descending aorta. (**b**) A left aortic arch with an aberrant right subclavian artery emanating from a diverticulum of Kommerell. The aberrant right subclavian artery forms a vascular ring by coursing posteriorly to its normal position. A cartoon of this anomaly and how it forms is depicted in Fig. 6.49a

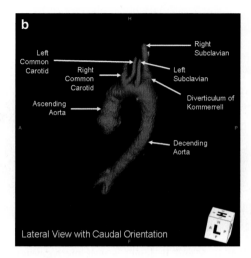

Fig. 6.49 (continued)

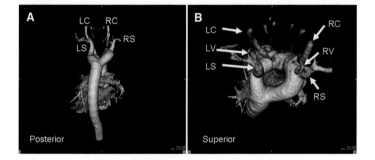

Fig. 6.50 Another example of a double aortic arch seen from the posterior (Panel A) and superior (Panel B) orientations in a baby. *LC* left carotid artery, *RC* right carotid artery, *LS* left subclavian artery, *RS* right subclavian artery, *LV* left vertebral artery, *RV* right vertebral artery. (Image provided courtesy of Russel Hirsch, MD, Assistant Professor and Director of the Cardiac Catheterization Laboratory, Cincinnati Children's Medical Center, Cincinnati, Ohio)

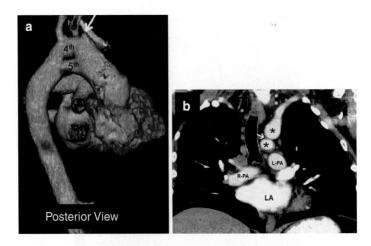

Fig. 6.51 Panels A and B depict a systemic to systemic type of persistent fifth branchial arch anomaly. Panel A is a volume-rendered, segmented example viewed from the posterior. "4th" demonstrates the normal aortic arch that forms from the fourth branchial arch. "5th" depicts the systemic to systemic anomalous fifth branchial arch connection. The *white arrow* depicts the right brachiocephalic artery near which the anomaly emanates. Panel B is a multiplanar reformat in axial plane depicting the typical double lumen aorta separated by periaortic fat which distinguishes this benign anomaly from an aortic dissection. (Reproduced with the kind permission of Elsevier.   Copyright 2009. Kligerman S, Blum A and Abbara S. Persistent fifth aortic arch in a patient with a history of intrauterine thalidomide exposure. *J Cardiovasc Comput Tomogr.* 2009;3:412–414)

aberrant right subclavian and right ligamentum arteriosum. If the ligamentum arteriosum is left sided in this latter anomaly, an incomplete ring would result.

Examples of incomplete vascular rings include an anomalous innominate artery, an aberrant right subclavian artery with a left-sided ligamentum arteriosum, and an anomalous left pulmonary artery (pulmonary vascular sling). The aberrant right subclavian artery (Fig. 6.49a, b) occurs in 0.1% of the population and is often asymptomatic. It arises from the

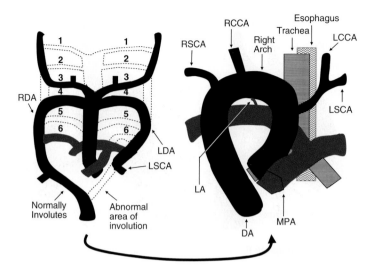

Fig. 6.52 A cartoon depicting the fetal development of a right aortic arch with no ring. Note the abnormal area of involution of the left dorsal aorta that causes this aberrancy. The distal portion of the right dorsal aorta remains. Numbers 1–6 represent the paired branchial arches. Dotted lines represent involution. *RDA* right dorsal aorta, *LDA* left dorsal aorta, *LSCA* left subclavian artery, *RSCA* right subclavian artery, *RCCA* right common carotid artery, *LCCA* left common carotid artery, *AA* ascending aorta, *LA* ligamentum arteriosum, *DA* descending aorta, *MPA* main pulmonary artery

descending aorta or from a Kommerell's diverticulum and crosses behind the esophagus and occurs when the fourth aortic arch and the right dorsal aorta involute above the seventh intersegmental artery.[131]

An anomalous innominate artery occurs when the innominate artery arises from the left side of the aortic arch. It may be asymptomatic or may result in respiratory symptoms when tracheal compression occurs.

Figure 6.55 illustrates a fine example of a hypoplastic aortic arch.

The anomalous left pulmonary artery (pulmonary vascular sling) occurs when the left pulmonary artery emanates from

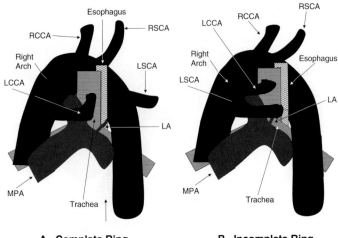

A. Complete Ring   **B. Incomplete Ring**

Fig. 6.53 A cartoon depicting a mirror image right aortic arch with both a complete and incomplete ring. Note the location of the ligamentum arteriosum (LA) attachments, which determines if the vascular ring is complete or incomplete. *LCCA* left common carotid artery, *RCCA* right common carotid artery, *RSCA* right subclavian artery, *LSCA* left subclavian artery, *MPA* main pulmonary artery

the right pulmonary artery and courses behind the trachea and in front of the esophagus to enter the hilum of the left lung (Fig. 6.42a, b) and results from the involution of the proximal left sixth branchial arch.[131] Normally, the proximal portions of the right and left sixth arch form the proximal right and left pulmonary arteries, respectively. The distal portion of the left sixth arch forms the ductus arteriosus and the distal part of the right sixth arch involutes. Buds from the sixth arch arteries grow into primitive lungs and connect to the primitive pulmonary circulation.

A patent ductus arteriosus results from failure of the ductus to close after birth (Fig. 6.56). Absence of a pulmonary artery may be due to abnormal involution of the proximal sixth arch on the affected side. The blood supply to the lung would then come from the bronchial arteries or from an ipsilateral patent ductus arteriosus.

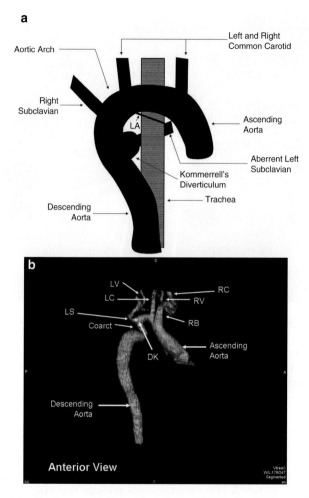

Fig. 6.54 (**a**) A cartoon depicting a right aortic arch with a complete vascular ring formed by the anomalous left subclavian artery emanating from a diverticulum of Kommerell and coursing posteriorly. The ring is completed by the connection of the ligamentum arteriosum (LA) to the aberrant left subclavian artery. (**b**) Three-dimensional, segmented reconstruction of a right aortic arch with an aberrant left subclavian artery forming a vascular ring as drawn in Fig. 6.53. In this example, a coarctation of the aorta (coarct) is present. *LS* left subclavian artery, *LC* left carotid artery, *LV* left vertebral artery, *RC* right carotid artery, *RV* right vertebral artery, DK diverticulum of Kommerell

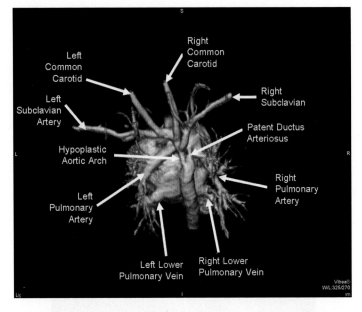

Fig. 6.55 An example of a hypoplastic arch from a baby. The image is a segmented, volume-rendered reconstruction. (Image provided courtesy of Russel Hirsch, MD, Assistant Professor and Director of the Cardiac Catheterization Laboratory, Cincinnati Childrens Medical Center, Cincinnati, Ohio)

6.2.7.2 Great Veins

The formation of the great veins is best understood if they are divided into two groups: the parietal veins and the visceral veins (Fig. 6.57). The visceral veins include the two vitelline veins and the two umbilical veins, which together open into the sinus venosus. The vitelline veins run on either side of the intestinal canal. They unite and are connected to each other by two anastomotic branches, one on the ventral and one on the dorsal side of the intestinal canal. Thus, the intestinal canal is circled by two vascular rings. The portions of the veins cephalad to the upper ring are interrupted by the developing liver and form sinusoids. The branches bringing blood

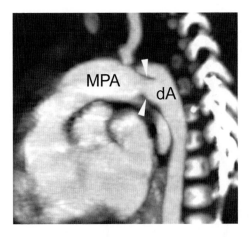

Fig. 6.56 A thick maximum intensity projection of a patent ductus arteriosus (*white arrow heads*) in a baby. *MPA* main pulmonary artery, *dA* descending aorta. (Reproduced with kind permission from Radiological Society of North America. Copyright 2003. Woo Goo H, Park IS, KonKo J, et al. CT of congenital heart disease: normal anatomy and typical pathologic conditions. *Radiographics*. 2003;23:S147–S165)

to these sinusoids are called the venae advehentes, which become the branches of the portal vein. The branches draining into the sinus venosus are called the venae revehentes and form the future hepatic veins. The left and right venae revehentes eventually connect. The remaining part of the upper venous ring forms the trunk of the portal vein.[131]

The two umbilical veins fuse to form a single trunk but remain separate. The right umbilical and vitelline veins disappear and the left umbilical and vitelline veins persist in utero. A branch ultimately forms between the upper venous ring and the right hepatic veins and forms the ductus venosus. The left umbilical vein and the ductus venosus involute after birth and form the ligamentum teres and ligamentum vensosum of the liver, respectively.[131]

Two short veins which open on either side of the sinus venosus form the beginning portion of the parietal system

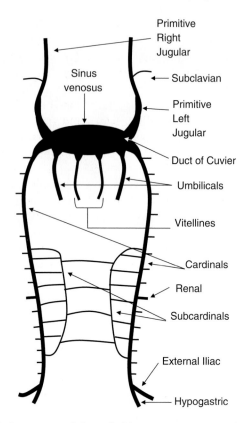

Fig. 6.57 A cartoon of the primitive venous anatomy in the fetus. See text for details.

and are called the ducts of Cuvier. Into each of these ducts empties an ascending and descending vein. The ascending veins return blood from below and are called the cardinal veins. The descending veins drain the head and are called the primitive jugular veins. The bilateral iliac and hypogastric veins drain blood from the primitive legs into the bilateral cardinal veins.[131]

The left cardinal vein below the left renal vein atrophies and the portion above the left renal vein remains as the hemi-azygous and accessory hemiazygous veins. The right cardinal vein now connects to both primitive limbs and eventually forms the lower portion of the inferior vena cava. Above the renal veins, the right cardinal vein becomes the azygos vein and transverse branches connect to it from the hemiazygous and accessory hemiazygous veins.[131]

The remainder of the inferior vena cava forms via the subcardinal veins. These veins lie parallel and ventral to the cardinal veins and initially have longitudinal anastomoses with the cardinal veins. The connection between the two subcardinal veins eventually disappears and is replaced by a single transverse vein at the level of the renal veins. The cross connections fuse into a single channel forming the rest of the inferior vena cava. The remaining portions involute.

The inferior vena cava at this level is formed by the proximal part of the ductus venosus, the prerenal part of the right subcardinal vein, the postrenal part of the right cardinal vein, and the cross branch which joins the two subcardinal veins. With the exception of a small portion of the left subcardinal vein which forms a suprarenal branch, the left subcardinal vein disappears.[131]

In contrast, the primitive jugular veins enlarge as the head develops. They also receive blood from the subclavian veins. The Cuvierian ducts are initially called the right and left superior venae cavae. A transverse branch develops (the innominate vein) and allows the two primitive jugular veins to connect. The section of the right primitive jugular vein between the left innominate vein and azygos vein forms the upper portion of the superior vena cava (SVC). The lower portion of the SVC is formed by the right Cuvierian duct. The left primitive jugular vein below the innominate vein and the left Cuvierian duct atrophies and disappears. Figure 6.58a, b depicts the fetal development of the great veins.

A double superior vena cava (SVC) forms if the transverse channel fails to connect the two primitive jugular veins. Thus, the left-sided SVC persists and drains into the right atrium via the coronary sinus. A single left-sided SVC emptying into the coronary sinus may occur if a vascular channel develops but the proximal part of the primitive jugular vein regresses.[131]

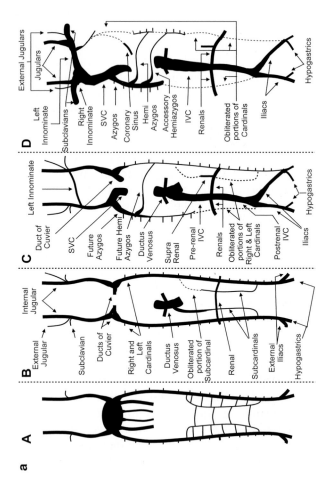

Fig. 6.58 (a) Cartoons depicting the fetal development of the great cardiac veins. (b) Cartoons depicting the fetal development of the great cardiac veins

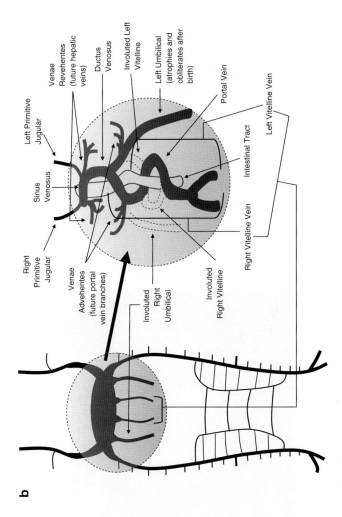

b

Fig. 6.58 (continued)

Figures 6.59–6.62 demonstrate examples of great vein anomalies.

6.3 Accuracy of Thoracic Aorta CT Angiography

Multidetector CT angiography (MDCT) is the mainstay for diagnosing most thoracic vascular abnormalities. It can detect various acute and chronic disorders including aortic aneurysm, pseudoaneurysm, aortic dissection, intramural hematoma, penetrating atherosclerotic ulcer, traumatic injury, rupture, inflammatory disorders, and congenital malformations.

CT has many advantages including its wide spread availability and its ability to image the vessel wall. In addition, it can identify anatomic anomalies and variants and branch vessel involvement of disease. Finally, it may distinguish among

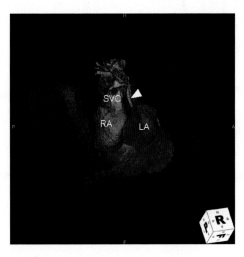

Fig. 6.59 An aberrant right superior vena cava (SVC) (*white arrow head*) entering the left atrium (LA). *RA* right atrium. The image is a semitransparent, segmented, volume-rendered reconstruction

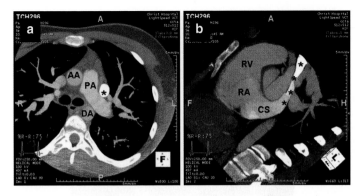

Fig. 6.60 A persistent left superior vena cava (*black asterisks*). This is a common great venous anomaly where the persistent superior vena cava usually empties into the coronary sinus (CS) which, as in this case, is dilated. Panel a is an axial thin maximum intensity projection (MIP). Panel b is a thick MIP in an oblique plane. *PA* pulmonary artery, *AA* ascending aorta, *DA* descending aorta, *RA* right atrium, *RV* right ventricle

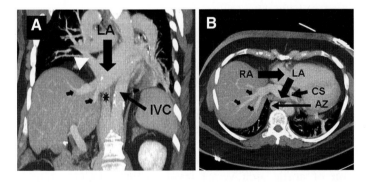

Fig. 6.61 Thick maximum intensity projections demonstrating total anomalous drainage of the hepatic veins (*small black arrows*) into the left atrium (LA). The black starburst in panel A is the azygous vein (AZ). Panel A is a coronal plane image and panel B is an axial plane image. *RA* right atrium, *CS* coronary sinus, *IVC* inferior vena cava. (Reproduced with kind permission from Elsevier. Copyright 2007. Kirsch J, Araoz P, Breen J, et al. Isolated total anomalous connection of the hepatic veins to the left atrium. *J Cardiovasc Comput Tomogr.* 2007;1:55–57)

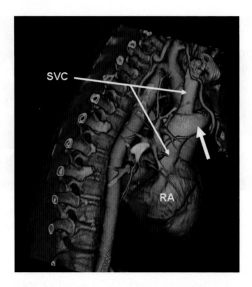

Fig. 6.62 Representation of a volume-rendered segmented image of an anomalous connection of a persistent left superior vena cava (*thick white arrow*) to the right superior vena cava. *RA* right atrium

the various acute aortic emergencies such as dissection, intramural hematoma, penetrating ulcer, and aortic rupture.

In two reports of 162 and 110 patients, respectively, the sensitivity of standard CT angiography for the diagnosis of aortic dissection was 83% and 98%, respectively, while the specificity was 87% and 100%, respectively.[138, 139] The accuracy of CT angiography appears to be substantially improved with helical multislice CT.[140–143] Spiral CT angiography may be more accurate than MR angiography or TEE in the detection of aortic arch vessel involvement.[140] ECG gating is required for accurate diagnosis to avoid motion artifact in the ascending aorta.[144, 145] The necessary cost for ECG gating is increased radiation exposure.

CT advantages include its availability in most hospitals on an emergency basis and its ability to identify intraluminal thrombus and pericardial effusion. Disadvantages include poor visualization of the intimal flap, seen <75% of the time, and rare identification of the entry site.[146] In addition, iodinated contrast may cause nephrotoxicity (gadolinium is also contraindicated in renal failure due to the risk of nephrogenic systemic fibrosis). Finally, aortic insufficiency is difficult to identify and quantify by CT.

CT is also accurate in confirming and characterizing aneurysms for exact location and extent. In addition, CT may be used to measure aortic diameters (arterial short axis), to identify complications (rupture, mycotic aneurysms, aortoenteric fistulas, etc.), and to follow aneurysms longitudinally. Finally, CT is useful for postprocedural surveillance after surgery and endovascular treatment.

6.4 Approach to Reading Thoracic Aorta CT Angiography

When performing a CT angiogram for the thoracic aorta, be sure to include a precontrast scan to detect subtle intramural hematoma as well as a contrasted scan and a delayed scan to evaluate for slow extravasation.

A systematic approach to reading thoracic CT angiograms is most useful. Similar to carotid CT, first assess the scan quality and contrast timing and opacity. A survey of the three-dimensional (3-D) data set is then recommended to survey the anatomy and to identify potential trouble spots. Again, diagnoses are never made from the 3-D data alone as these images are prone to error. After the general 3-D survey, maximum intensity projection (MIP) images in axial and longitudinal planes are examined in detail. All major arteries are visually traced systematically. Begin with the aorta and follow it to the caudal limit of the scan. Trace the visualized portions of the arch vessels and any major descending aortic branches.

Curved multiplanar reformatting (cMPR) may be utilized in difficult to trace arterial segments. MPR is employed to visualize diseased locations in more detail and to finalize specific pathologic diagnoses.

As with all vascular CT analyses, the atherosclerotic burden, calcification, and stenosis grade are assessed. Aneurysms are identified and detailed measurements are made in the true axial and longitudinal planes (may often be off-axis planes) and centerline measurements are made to characterize the aneurysm, especially if percutaneous stenting is contemplated. Mural thrombus is noted.

Dissections are excluded. Aortic dissection may be diagnosed by CT angiography if two distinct lumens with a visible intimal flap can be identified. The CT scan should classify the dissection (Debakey or Stanford), localize the tear, identify the true versus false lumen, identify whether the important branch vessels emanate from the true or false lumen, identify arch involvement, and identify thrombus. Pericardial fluid and aortic rupture may also be identified. Old dissection may be differentiated from acute dissection as the contrast in the false lumen of a chronic dissection is less dense due to more mature thrombosis.

Anomalies are characterized and described. Ancillary findings should be identified if present.

Reporting should be organized, concise, and clinically relevant. The 2010 guidelines for the diagnosis and management of patients with thoracic aortic disease list the essential elements of aortic imaging reports and these are depicted in Table 6.6.[28] In addition, techniques to minimize radiation are recommended and discussed in a previous chapter. Finally, relating aortic diameter to the patient's age, body size, and gender is recommended if possible (see Tables 6.1–6.2).

Chapter 7
Abdominal Aortic CT Angiography

7.1 Anatomy (Figs. 7.1–7.4)

The abdominal aorta begins at the aortic hiatus of the diaphragm and terminates at the aortic bifurcation to become the iliac arteries. Abdominal aortic branches are divided into three sets: visceral, parietal, and terminal branches. Visceral branches

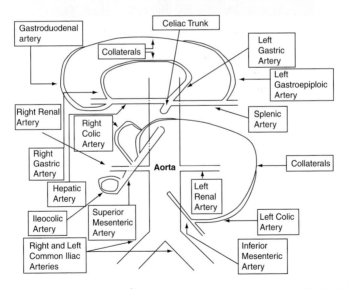

FIGURE 7.1. A cartoon illustrating the anatomy of the abdominal aorta, its branches, and its anastomoses.

R. Pelberg, W. Mazur, *Vascular CT Angiography Manual*,
DOI: 10.1007/978-1-84996-260-5_7,
© Springer-Verlag London Limited 2011

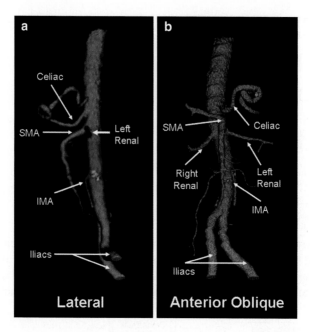

FIGURE 7.2. A volume-rendered, segmented reconstruction of the abdominal aorta and its branches. Panel a is volume rendered, segmented lateral projection image. Panel b is an anterior view of the same. SMA: Superior mesenteric artery. IMA: Inferior mesenteric artery. Celiac: Celiac trunk. Left renal: Left renal artery. Right renal: Right renal artery.

include the celiac artery, the superior mesenteric artery (SMA), the inferior mesenteric artery (IMA), the middle suprarenal arteries, the renal arteries, the internal spermatic arteries, and the ovarian arteries (in females). With the exception of the SMA and IMA, all visceral branches are paired. Parietal branches include the inferior phrenic arteries (paired), the lumbar arteries (paired), and the middle sacral artery. The common iliac arteries make up the terminal branches.

The celiac artery is a short trunk arising from the anterior aorta just below the diaphragm and divides into the left gastric artery, the hepatic artery, and the splenic artery. Rarely, the hepatic and splenic arteries arise directly from the aorta (Fig. 7.5).

The left gastric artery distributes branches to the esophagus which connects with the aortic esophageal arteries. The

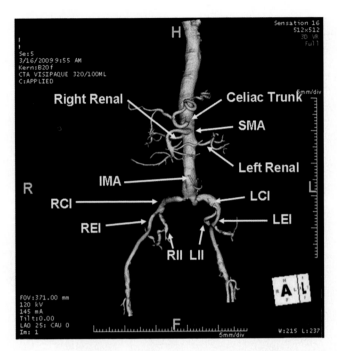

FIGURE 7.3. An anterior volume-rendered depiction of the abdominal aorta and its major branches. Right renal: Right renal artery. Left renal: Left renal artery. SMA: Superior mesenteric artery. IMA: Inferior mesenteric artery. RCI: Right common iliac artery. LCI: Left common iliac artery. REI: Right external iliac artery. LEI: Left external iliac artery. RII: Right internal (hypogastric) iliac artery. LII: Left internal iliac (hypogastric) artery.

left gastric artery then supplies the lesser curvature of the stomach and forms an anastomosis with the right gastric artery. The hepatic artery supplies the superior part of the duodenum and then supplies the lesser omentum. It then supplies the lobes of the liver. Branches of the hepatic artery include the right gastric artery and the gastroduodenal artery. The gastroduodenal artery forms the right gastroepiploic artery and the pancreaticoduodenal artery, which then supplies the stomach, pancreas, and duodenum.

The right gastric artery supplies part of the lesser curvature of the stomach and forms an anastomosis with the left gastric artery. The tortuous splenic artery supplies the spleen,

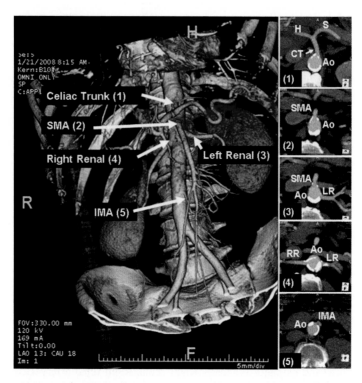

FIGURE 7.4. Depiction of the normal abdominal aorta anatomy. The color image is a volume-rendered reconstruction of the abdominal aorta. The gray-scale images to the right represent maximum intensity projections (MIP) at various axial planes corresponding to the major abdominal aorta branches labeled (1) to (5). Image (1) is at the level of the celiac trunk (CT) and demonstrates the branching of the hepatic (H) and splenic (S) arteries. Image (2) shows the superior mesenteric artery (SMA) take off. Image (3) shows the take off of the left renal artery (LR) which is more superior in this case than the right renal artery (RR) shown in image (4). Image (5) depicts the small inferior mesenteric artery (IMA) branch point. Ao: Aorta.

pancreas, and stomach. Its branches are the pancreatic artery, the short gastric artery, and the left gastroepiploic artery. The left gastroepiploic artery runs the greater curvature of the stomach and connects with the right gastroepiploic artery. It also forms an anastomosis with the middle colic artery.

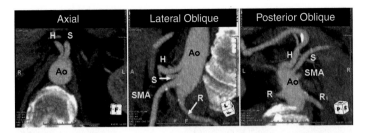

FIGURE 7.5. Illustration of an example from a patient with a separate take off of the hepatic (H) and splenic (S) arteries arising directly from the aorta (Ao). The celiac trunk is absent. SMA: Superior mesenteric artery. R: Renal artery.

The SMA supplies the entire small intestines except the superior duodenum. It also supplies the cecum, the ascending colon, and half of the transverse colon. It moves downward and forward forming an anastomotic network with various intestinal and colonic branches via the left middle colic, the right middle colic, and the ileocolic arteries. The SMA connects to the IMA via the left colic artery and forms an anastomosis with itself via the ileocolic artery.

The IMA supplies the left half of the transverse colon, the descending colon, and a significant portion of the rectum. IMA branches include the left colic artery, the sigmoid artery, and the superior hemorrhoidal artery, which supplies the remainder of the rectum.

At their periphery, the middle colic, right colic, and ileocolic arteries may form an interconnection that courses to the junction of the transverse and descending colon. This connection is termed the arc of Riolan or the wandering artery of Drummond (Fig. 7.6). The arc of Riolan may be hypertrophied in cases of mesenteric ischemia as is the case in Fig. 7.6. The wandering artery of Drummond will anastomose with the left colic artery, a branch of the IMA. Cecal branches also arise from the ileocolic branch.

The arc of Riolan provides the primary source of collateral blood flow between the SMA and the IMA. Other sources of collateral circulation involve the anastomoses of the internal mammary artery and the inferior epigastric artery and the

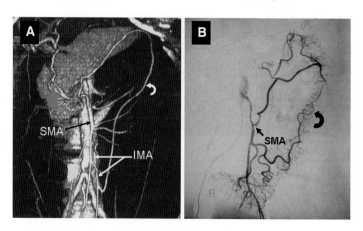

FIGURE 7.6. Demonstration of the arc of Riolan or the wandering artery of Drummond (*black and white curved arrows*). Panel A is a volume-rendered, semitransparent computed tomography (CT) angiographic image and panel B is an invasive angiogram. The arc of Riolan is the main source of collaterals between the superior mesenteric artery (SMA) and the inferior mesenteric artery (IMA) (Reproduced with kind permission from Radiological Society of North America. Kirkpatrick I, Kroeker M, Greenberg H. Biphasic CT with mesenteric CT angiography in the evaluation of acute mesenteric ischemia: initial experience. *Radiology*. 2003;229:91–98).

communication between the SMA, the IMA, and the internal pudendal arteries. In addition, the lumbar arteries form an anastomosis with the hypogastric artery.

7.2 Disease Processes

7.2.1 Atherosclerosis of the Abdominal Aorta and Its Branches

Significant obstruction of the intestinal arteries has been noted in 6–10% of unselected autopsies and in 14–24% of patients undergoing abdominal arteriography.[185] Since intestinal ischemia is rare, however, there are no good studies regarding its true prevalence and natural history. Because of extensive mesenteric artery collateralization, intestinal artery obstruction is often asymptomatic. As with all vascular diseases, the most common pathology in the abdominal aorta and its branches is atherosclerosis. Other far less common etiologies include degenerative disorders such as Marfan's and Ehlers–Danlos syndrome, fibromuscular dysplasia (FMD), and vasculitis.

Acute intestinal ischemia most commonly results from obstruction and more rarely from low flow. Causes of obstruction may include acute thrombosis or embolism. Nearly two-thirds of patients with acute intestinal ischemia are women aged 70 and above.[186-188] Mesenteric artery stenosis is strongly associated with advancing age and with the presence of coronary artery disease (CAD).[186] Without treatment, acute intestinal ischemia is uniformly fatal.

Chronic intestinal ischemia is almost always due to atherosclerosis.[185] Rare causes include FMD and Buerger's disease.[190] Patients are most often female.[191, 182]

Figures 7.7–7.11 are examples of etiologies of both acute and chronic mesenteric ischemia. Figures 7.12–7.14 depict examples of complete abdominal aortic occlusion.

7.2.2 Celiac Compression Syndrome

The median arcuate ligament of the diaphragm is formed by muscular fibers that connect the right and left crura of the diaphragm, and defines the anterior margin of the aortic hiatus. Compression of the celiac axis by this ligament is referred to as celiac artery compression syndrome or median arcuate ligament syndrome, and has been reported to cause intestinal angina (Figs. 7.15a,b and 7.16).[199, 194] While surgical treatment can lead to persistent clinical improvement in symptomatic patients,[194] the importance of celiac artery compression in asymptomatic patients is unknown.[195]

Results of conventional angiographic studies dating to the early 1970s demonstrate that the positions of the median arcuate ligament, celiac artery, and aorta vary considerably during respiration. Median arcuate ligament compression is often accentuated during expiration.[196, 197] The diagnosis of celiac compression syndrome may be made by dynamic invasive angiography. Celiac artery compression is noted during expiration and disappears during inspiration. The diagnosis is more difficult by CT angiography since dynamic studies are more difficult to perform and the ligament itself may be difficult to visualize on CT. A clue to the CT diagnosis is that no atherosclerosis or other cause of a celiac artery stenosis is identified.

FIGURE 7.7. An example of chronic atherosclerotic mesenteric ischemia. Panel A illustrates the volume-rendered image of all mesenteric vessels demonstrating the full anatomic relationships. Panel B is a volume-rendered, segmented image of the mesenteric vessels only. There is a severe stenosis of the ileocolic artery (*arrowhead*). In addition, there are high-grade stenoses of the celiac trunk (Celiac) and the superior mesenteric artery (SMA) depicted by their labeled arrows. The *dashed arrow* points out the hypertrophied arc of Riolan which further serves to demonstrate the degree of chronic ischemia. Chronic atherosclerotic mesenteric ischemia requires significant stenoses of at least two of the major mesenteric arteries. Recall that stenoses are not diagnosed by volume-rendered imaging alone, which is used for general anatomic evaluation. Maximum intensity projections (MIP) and multiplanar reformatting (MPR) are used to confirm the presence of a stenosis. As noted in panels C and D, the MPR demonstrates high-grade stenoses (*arrows*) of the celiac trunk and the SMA. IMA: Inferior mesenteric artery (Reproduced with kind permission of Springer. Copyright 2008. Cademartiri F, Palumbo A, Maffei E, et al. Noninvasive evaluation of the celiac trunk and superior mesenteric artery with multislice CT in patients with chronic mesenteric ischemia. *La Radiologica Medica*. 2008;113:1135–1142).

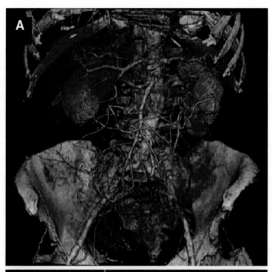

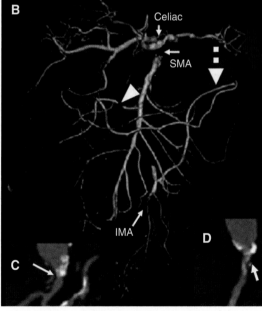

7.2.3 Nutcracker Syndrome

The nutcracker syndrome is caused by a rare congenital abnormality. It results from compression of the left renal vein and can occur in one of two ways. The renal vein may be compressed either by the SMA arising from the aorta in an acute angle or by a posterior coursing renal vein behind the aorta. If the renal vein is located posterior to the aorta, it may be compressed between the aorta and the vertebrae, and may result in hydronephrosis and ultimately in renal insufficiency. This syndrome occurs more commonly in women and presents by the third or fourth decades. Treatment is usually conservative though stenting, venous embolization, or surgery can be performed. Figure 7.17a and b demonstrate the two forms of nutcracker syndrome.

7.2.4 Aneurysms

7.2.4.1 Abdominal Aorta

Abdominal aortic aneurysm (AAA) (Figs. 7.18–7.24) is defined as a dilation of the abdominal aorta to ≥50% of the proximal normal segment or to an absolute diameter of ≥3 cm.[143] The normal abdominal aorta diameters in males and

Figure 7.8. Depiction of curved multiplanar reformats (cMPR) of varying degrees of stenoses in various splanchnic vessels. Panel A shows a normal superior mesenteric artery (SMA). Panel B demonstrates a calcified SMA without significant obstruction. Panel C illustrates a nonsignificant stenosis of the celiac trunk. Panel D displays a significant SMA stenosis with a mixed plaque (calcified and noncalcified). Panel E depicts a subtotal occlusion of the SMA and panel F demonstrates an occluded SMA (Reproduced with kind permission of Springer. Copyright 2008. Cademartiri F, Palumbo A, Maffei E, et al. Noninvasive evaluation of the celiac trunk and superior mesenteric artery with multislice CT in patients with chronic mesenteric ischemia. *Radiol Med*. 2008;113:1135–1142).

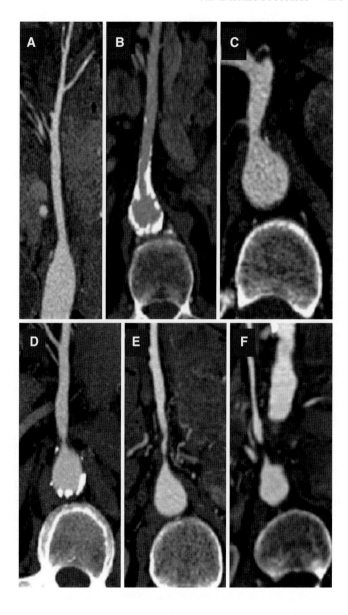

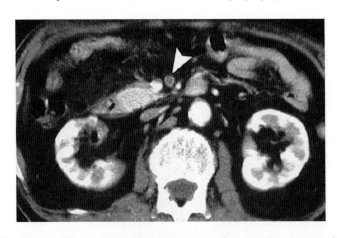

FIGURE 7.9. Illustration of an embolus to the superior mesenteric artery (SMA) (*arrowhead*) demonstrated by the filling defect within the artery surrounded by a thin ring of contrast enhancement, resulting in acute mesenteric ischemia (Reproduced with kind permission from the American Roentgen Ray Society. Copyright 2009. Furukawa A, Kanasaki S, Kono N, et al. CT diagnosis of acute mesenteric ischemia from various causes. *Am J Roentgenol*. 2009;192:408–416).

females are 2.1 ± 0.2 cm and 1.53 ± 0.22 cm, respectively. The average growth rate of an AAA is 0.3–0.4 cm per year and the natural history is that of expansion and eventual rupture. If growth is more accelerated, impending rupture must be considered.

The overall prevalence of AAA ranges from 4% to 8% in men and approximately 1% in women.[144, 145] However, the true prevalence of AAA varies with patient demographics and increases in prevalence with age, male gender, and family history of AAA.[146] The annual incidence of AAA has been reported to be 40–50 per 100,000 men and 7–12 per 100,000 women.[147] Aneurysms are systemic and thus identification of an AAA mandates a search for aneurysms in other parts of the aorta.

Most aortic and peripheral aneurysms result from medial degeneration most frequently due to atherosclerosis. Connective tissue abnormalities resulting from congenital diseases such as

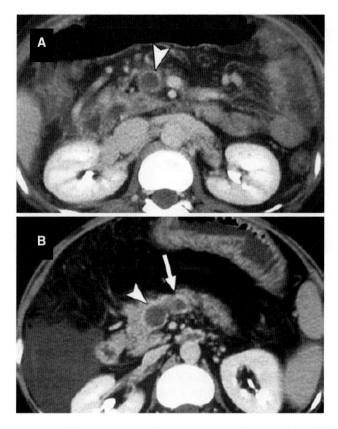

FIGURE 7.10. Demonstration of two examples of thrombosis of the superior mesenteric vein resulting in mesenteric ischemia. Panel A demonstrates a filling defect in the superior mesenteric vein (*arrowhead*). Panel B from another patient shows the same (*arrowhead*). It also depicts the typical bowel thickening and enhancement noted when ischemic bowel is present (*arrow*) (Reproduced with kind permission from the American Roentgen Ray Society. Copyright 2009. Furukawa A, Kanasaki S, Kono N, et al. CT diagnosis of acute mesenteric ischemia from various causes. *Am J Roentgenol.* 2009;192:408–416).

Marfan's syndrome and Ehlers–Danlos syndrome may also result in aneurysm formation. Another rare and unique cause of AAA is the inflammatory AAA. These are associated with thick,

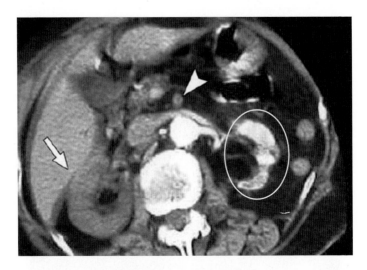

FIGURE 7.11. Depiction of a maximum intensity projection (MIP), axial image of an embolism to the superior mesenteric artery (SMA) (*arrowhead*). Of note, there is no contrast enhancement of the right kidney (*arrow*), indicating that an embolus has also occluded the right renal artery. The left kidney (*circled*) does enhance indicating there is blood flow to this kidney (Reproduced with kind permission from the American Roentgen Ray Society. Copyright 2009. Furukawa A, Kanasaki S, Kono N, et al. CT diagnosis of acute mesenteric ischemia from various causes. *Am J Roentgenol*. 2009;192:408–416).

fibrotic aortic walls[148] and elevated sedimentation rates. They have been shown to be present in up to 4.5% of those presenting for elective AAA repair.[149] More than 90% of patients with inflammatory AAAs are smokers.[149] Finally, primary aortic wall infections are another very rare cause of AAA.

The four most important risk factors for the development of an AAA are age ≥65 years, male gender, cigarette smoking, and family history of AAA in a first-degree relative. Secondary predisposing factors include hypertension, hyperlipidemia, and established cardiovascular disease.[147, 150] Risk factors predisposing to AAA expansion are age ≥70 years, renal transplant, cardiac transplant, previous stroke, severe cardiac disease, and tobacco use.[151]

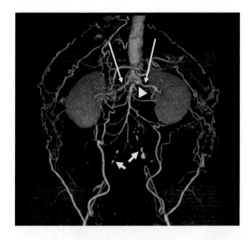

FIGURE 7.12. Demonstration of a complete occlusion of the aorta (*white arrowhead*) just distal to the renal arteries (*long white arrows*). The leg vessels are supplied by a vast array of collaterals that hypertrophied over time. The *short white arrows* demonstrate the calcific casts of the iliac arteries. The image is a segmented, semi-transparent, volume-rendered reconstruction (Reproduced with kind permission from H M P Communications. Copyright 2009. Bhamidipati C, Amankwah K, Costanza M. Chronic mesenteric ischemia with aortic occlusion. *Vasc Dis Manag.* 2009;6(7):26–27).

Those at increased risk for AAA rupture are patients with cardiac or renal transplant, female gender, uncontrolled hypertension, larger initial AAA diameter, and current tobacco use.[151] Other features predictive of AAA rupture include female gender (smaller aorta) and a focal discontinuity in the circumferential calcification.[152] The 1-year incidence of AAA rupture is 9% for aneurysms of 5.5–6 cm, 10% for aneurysms from 6 to 6.9 cm, and 33% for aneurysms ≥7 cm.[153] Another rarely seen but important sign of impending rupture is the hyperattenuated crescent sign (Fig. 7.25).[152, 154, 155] Visible only on the noncontrasted CT scan, the hyperattenuating crescent sign represents an acute intramural or mural thrombus hemorrhage and predicts impending rupture since the earliest stage of rupture begins with blood penetrating the margin of the mural thrombus. Finally, aneurysm shape

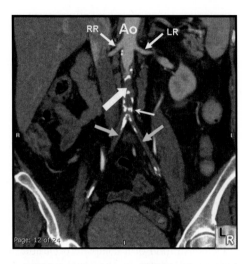

FIGURE 7.13. Multiplanar reformat (MPR) of an aortic occlusion distal to the renal arteries. RR: Right renal artery. LR: Left renal artery. Ao: Aorta. The *thick white arrow* demonstrates the diffuse thrombus within the aorta which is spotted with calcifications (*thin white arrow*). The *yellow arrows* point to the iliac arteries which are also thrombosed.

also predicts rupture. Saccular aneurysms rupture more frequently than fusiform aneurysms (Figs. 6.9 and 6.10).

Mortality rates after AAA rupture are 70–94% and up to 62% die before reaching hospital. Emergent surgical repair has a mortality rate of 50% compared to 4% for elective surgical repair in a stable AAA.[151]

Screening for AAA

A one-time screening exam is recommended for men and women ≥65 years who have ever smoked cigarettes or in whom a diagnosis of CAD is present. For men and women with a family history of AAA the initial screening age is lowered to ≥50 years. Screening is also recommended for men and women who have had coronary artery bypass grafting.[156] In addition, the presence of a popliteal or femoral artery

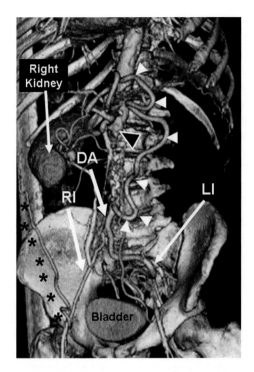

FIGURE 7.14. Demonstration of a volume-rendered reconstruction of a chronic aortic occlusion. The patient has undergone a left nephrectomy. The aortic occlusion point is demonstrated by the *black arrowhead*. There is an arc of Riolan (*white arrowheads*) collateralizing the distal aorta (DA). The *black asterisks* outline collaterals to the right iliac artery (RI). LI: Left iliac artery.

aneurysm should elicit a screen for AAA, since AAA is present in nearly 62% and 85% of patients with popliteal or femoral artery aneurysms, respectively.[151] Conversely, 14% of patients with AAA will have a femoral or popliteal aneurysm.[151]

Screening is usually performed by a one-time abdominal aortic ultrasound which has been shown to have a 95% sensitivity and a 100% specificity for detecting aneurysm $\geq$3 cm.[157] CT angiography and magnetic resonance imaging may be used if ultrasound is not optimal, but due to the radiation and iodinated contrast exposure these imaging examinations are reserved mainly for characterization before and follow-up after endovascular treatment. Physical examination alone has been shown to be ineffective.[158]

Once an AAA is detected, a surveillance program should be established. If no AAA is initially found, no further testing is necessary. Yearly screening is recommended for AAA between 3 and 4 cm. Surveillance every 6 months is required if the AAA is 4–5 cm.[156]

Treatment of AAA

Once an AAA is detected, three treatment options are available, including medical management only, endovascular aneurysm repair (EVAR) (Figure 7.26), and surgical repair. Medical management is mandatory for all aneurysms and should focus on secondary prevention with treatment for hypertension, dyslipidemia (AAA is a CAD equivalent), and smoking cessation. Beta-blockers are also indicated.

Accepted indications for intervention include size >5 cm, growth >0.5 cm per year, or when symptoms are present. While most AAAs are detected serendipitously, symptoms

---

FIGURE 7.15. (a) Depiction of a beautiful example of a patient with celiac compression syndrome (*arrowheads*) caused by compression of the celiac trunk by the arcuate ligament. Panels A and B are volume-rendered reconstructions. Panel C is a maximum intensity projection (MIP) and panel D is a multiplanar reformat (MPR). Note the compression of the celiac artery in panels A to C with no evidence of atherosclerotic plaque. Panel D demonstrates the arcuate ligament crossing the celiac axis. SMA: Superior mesenteric artery. Ao: Aorta. Celiac: Celiac artery. (Images courtesy of Sanjay Srivatsa MD, FACC. Innovis Health, Fargo, ND.) (b) A three-dimensional reconstruction of the plane of compression of the celiac axis from the patient depicted in (a). The arcuate ligament is well visualized crossing the celiac trunk. CT: Celiac trunk (Images courtesy of Sanjay Srivatsa MD, FACC. Innovis Health, Fargo, ND).

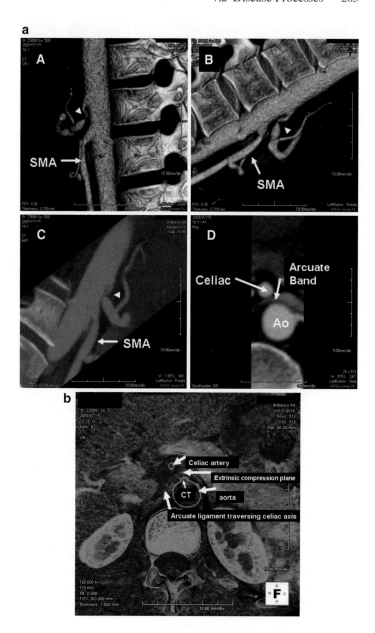

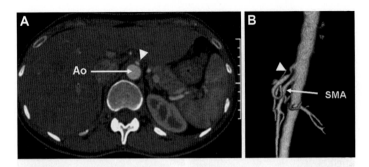

FIGURE 7.16. Another example of the celiac compression syndrome. Panel A is a multiplanar reformatted (MPR) axial image nicely demonstrating the compression of the celiac artery by the arcuate ligament (*white arrow head*). Panel B demonstrates the celiac artery compression (*white arrow head*) in a volume-rendered, segmented reconstruction. Ao: Aorta. SMA: Superior mesenteric artery (Reproduced with kind permission from Elsevier. Copyright 2007. Grierson C, Uberoi R, Warakaulle D. Multidetector CT appearances of splanchnic arterial pathology. *Clin Radiol.* 2007;62:717–723).

FIGURE 7.17. (**a**) A multiplanar reformatted (MPR) image of the nutcracker syndrome. In this example, the renal vein (*black asterisk*) is compressed between the superior mesenteric artery (SMA) and the aorta (Ao). The *black arrow* shows the compression of the vein and the *white arrow* shows the dilated vein proximal to the point of compression. (Reproduced with kind permission from Servier International. Copyright 2009. Image courtesy of Olivier Hartung, Marseille, France. Hartung H. Nutcracker syndrome. *Phlebolymphology.* 2009;16:246–252.) (**b**) The second variant of the nutcracker syndrome. Here, the left renal vein (*black arrowhead*) is compressed between the aorta and the spine. This is caused by the posterior course of the left renal vein behind the aorta (Ao) (*large black arrow*). The normal left renal vein course is anterior to the aorta (Reproduced with kind permission from Servier International. Copyright 2009. Image courtesy of Olivier Hartung, Marseille, France. Hartung H. Nutcracker syndrome. *Phlebolymphology.* 2009;16:246–252).

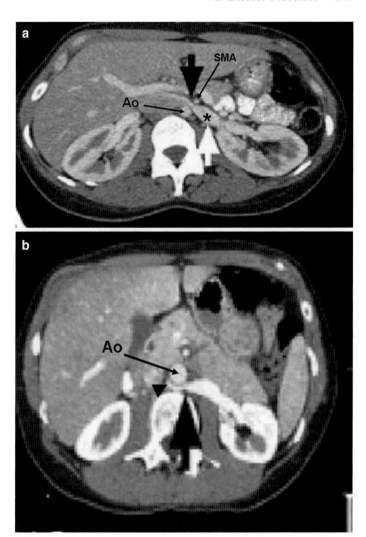

may include back pain and abdominal pain. Since anecdotal observations indicate that some aneurysms rupture at unusually small sizes while others grow to exceptionally large sizes without rupture, newer indications for intervention have

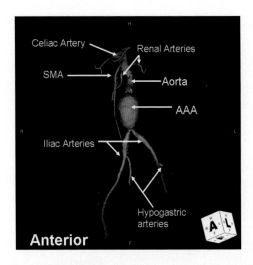

FIGURE 7.18. A nice example of an infrarenal, fusiform abdominal aortic aneurysm (AAA). SMA: Superior mesenteric artery.

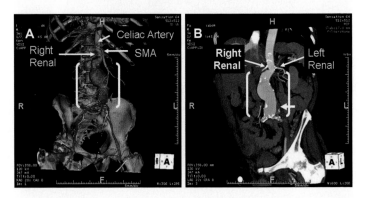

FIGURE 7.19. Depiction of a fusiform abdominal aortic aneurysm (AAA) (*bracketed*). Note the partial thrombosis (*white arrow* in panel B). Panel A is a volume-rendered reconstruction and panel B is a maximum intensity projection (MIP). The thrombus evident in panel B is not well appreciated on the volume-rendered image (panel A). The aneurysm begins below the renal arteries and extends to the iliac bifurcation. There is a stent in the ostial right renal artery (right renal). Left renal: Left renal artery. SMA: Superior mesenteric artery.

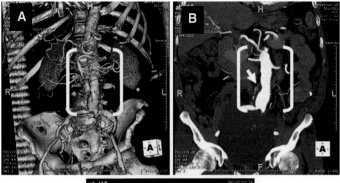

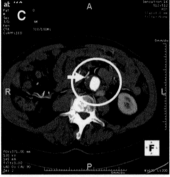

FIGURE 7.20. Illustration of a partially thrombosed aortic aneurysm (bracketed in panels A and B and circled in panel C). Panel A is a volume-rendered image and panels B and C are maximum intensity projections (MIP) in the anterior plane (panel B) and axial plane (panel C). Note the thrombus (*white arrow*) and the calcified outline of the arterial wall around the thrombus. The aneurysm is not obviously apparent on the volume-rendered image in panel A since the thrombosed sac does not fill with contrast.

been proposed and include sizes greater than 2.5 times the DAR (diameter of aorta at the renal arteries) and finite element analysis (FEA).

FEA is a mathematical model to characterize structural mechanics. It uses a system of simultaneous equations and assumptions to solve for deformation and stresses in dynamic

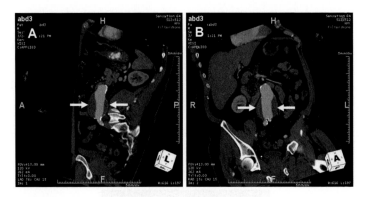

FIGURE 7.21. Demonstration of multiplanar reformatted (MPR) images depicting a saccular aneurysm in the distal abdominal aorta (between the *white arrows*). The aneurysm is thrombosed. Panel A is a lateral plane and panel B is an anterior plane.

structures by constructing geometrically similar models consisting of discrete regions called finite elements. After market computer programs can perform these analyses. By predicting rupture points and wall stresses better than diameter, some studies have shown FEA, using three-dimensional CT reconstructions, to be better than diameter for differentiating AAA rupture risk.[159, 160] Peak stress of an aneurysm is often, but not always, demonstrated at the aneurysm shoulder points.

When deciding to repair an AAA, the rupture risk must be weighed against the risk of repair in the context of life expectancy. Figure 7.27 proposes an algorithm to decide the optimal AAA treatment option. Whenever feasible, EVAR is often recommended. It involves placing a percutaneous stent into the AAA to exclude the aneurysm from aortic blood flow, to reduce the risk of rupture, and to ultimately decrease the diameter of the excluded aneurysm.

Multiple EVAR stent grafts are available on the market and their CT angiographic appearance is specific to the stent graft type. The type of stent graft used is mainly operator-dependent. The Vanguard (Boston Scientific/Scimed, Natick, Massachusetts) is a self-expanding graft with a nitinol framework covered with a Dacron fabric (Fig. 7.28).

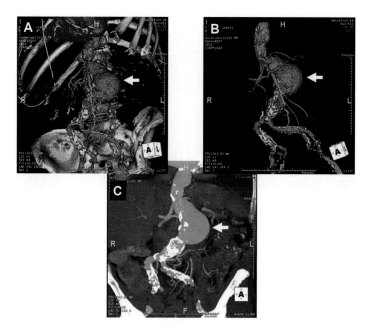

FIGURE 7.22. Another example of an abdominal aortic aneurysm (AAA) (*white arrows* in panels A, B, and C). Panel A is a volume-rendered reconstruction. Panel B is a segmented volume-rendered image, and panel C is a maximum intensity projection (MIP). Note the distorted, tortuous contour of the aorta resulting from the growth of the aneurysm.

The AneuRx (Medtronic, Santa Rosa, California) (Figs. 7.29, 7.30, and 6.13) is also a self-expanding, diamond-shaped, modular stent with nitinol elements that help secure it to the aortic wall with high radial force and no expanding hooks. It is made of a high-density, polyester graft material with low porosity. Its CT appearance is that of small diamonds.

Medtronic also makes a suprarenal stent graft called the Talent (World Medical/Medtronic, Sunrise, Florida) (Fig. 7.31). It consists of a woven polyester tube supported by a tubular metal web that expands to a pre-established diameter when placed in the artery. Because it is a suprarenal graft, its proximal apposition with the aorta occurs proximal

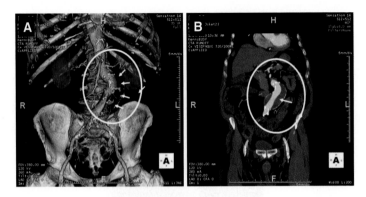

FIGURE 7.23. Demonstration of a volume-rendered reconstruction (panel A) and a maximum intensity projection (MIP) (panel B) of an infrarenal abdominal aortic aneurysm (AAA). Note the thrombus in panel B (*white arrow*) with the displaced calcium on the aortic wall. The thrombus is not well visualized on the three-dimensional image in panel A but a clue to its presence is given by the displaced calcium (*white arrows*).

to the renal arteries and thus the graft will span across the renal arteries. Since most stent grafts begin below the renal arteries, preceding knowledge of the placement of a Talent graft is necessary to avoid concern for proximal stent migration on post-EVAR surveillance imaging. The Talent stent graft has a "zig zag" appearance on CT image.

The Zenith stent graft (Cook, Bloomington, Indiana) (Figs. 7.32–7.34) is also a suprarenal graft and is composed of a modular, self-expanding stent made of a woven polyester graft material similar to that used in open surgical repair. Surgical suture is used to sew the graft material to the stainless steel stent frame. The graft's three parts include a "main body" and two "legs." The main body is positioned in the aorta. The legs are positioned in the iliac arteries and connected to the main body. Thus, the graft extends from the suprarenal aorta into both iliac arteries. The iliac extension pieces have flared ends to accommodate longer iliac arteries. On CT it also resembles large "zig zags."

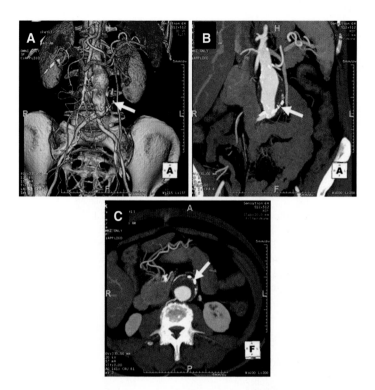

FIGURE 7.24. Another example of an abdominal aortic aneurysm (AAA). Panel A is a three-dimensional image where the size of the aneurysm is not well appreciated. However, displaced calcium is seen (*white arrow*) providing a clue to its size. It is more clearly depicted in panel B (maximum intensity projection [MIP], coronal plane) and panel C (MIP, axial plane). The *white arrows* in panels B and C also point to the displaced calcium in the aortic wall which surrounds the thrombosed aneurysm.

The Gore EXCLUDER AAA Endoprosthesis (W.L. Gore & Associates, Flagstaff, Arizona) (Figs. 7.35–7.37) is a bifur-cated, modular graft with an outer self-expanding nitinol sup-port structure and a low permeability film layer. The CT appearance of the Gore is similar to that of the Cook Zenith graft but the "zig zags" appear smaller and the graft begins in the infrarenal aorta.

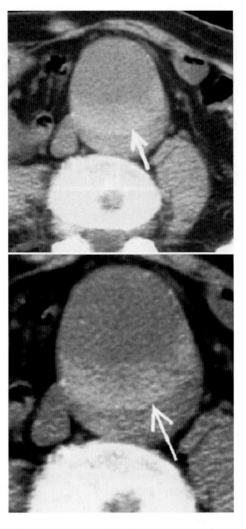

FIGURE 7.25. Demonstration of the hyperattenuated crescent sign, a clue to pending aortic rupture. This is a noncontrasted scan. See text for details (Reproduced with kind permission from the Radiological Society of North America. Copyright 1999. Gonsalves CF. The hyperattenuating crescent sign. *Radiology*. 1999;211:37–38).

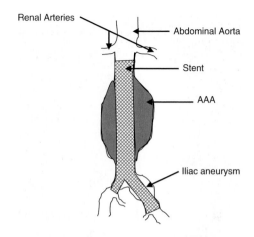

FIGURE 7.26. A cartoon depicting an endovascular stent for an abdominal aortic aneurysm (AAA).

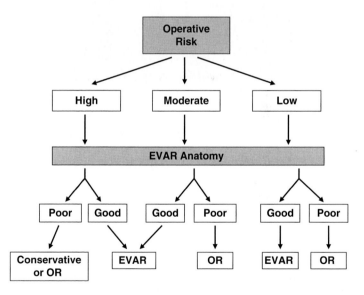

FIGURE 7.27. A logical decision tree for the treatment of an abdominal aortic aneurysm (AAA).

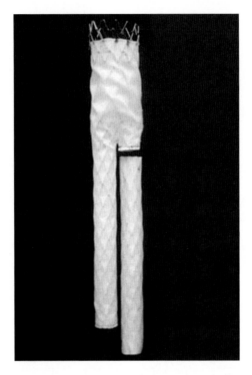

FIGURE 7.28. Depiction of the Vanguard endovascular stent graft (Boston Scientific/Scimed, Natick, Massachusetts) (Reproduced with kind permission from Springer. Copyright 2001. Diethrich E. AAA stent grafts: current developments. *J Invasive Cardiol.* 2001;13(5):1–13).

The Ancure stent graft (Guidant, Menlo Park, California) (Fig. 7.38) is a unibody, nonsupported woven polyester graft. It is available in tube, bifurcated, and aortoiliac options. The system incorporates four independent double hooks that penetrate the arterial wall for fixation. There are separate attachment systems available for the proximal and distal ends.

Finally, the Endologix Powerlink stent graft (Endologix, Irvine, California) (Fig. 7.39) is a one-piece, self-expanding

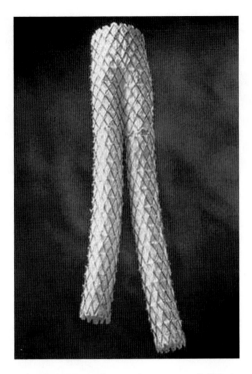

FIGURE 7.29. An AneuRx endovascular stent graft (Medtronic, Santa Rosa, California). The typical appearance on computed tomography (CT) is noted in Figs. 6.13 and 7.30 (Reproduced with kind permission from Springer. Copyright 2001. Dietrich E. AAA stent grafts: current developments. *J Invasive Cardiol.* 2001;13(5):1–13).

design supported by a cobalt–chromium alloy stent to reduce kinking. Since the graft fabric is attached to the stent skeleton at the proximal and distal ends only, the fabric of the graft balloons off of the stent cage during the cardiac cycle. This allows blood to flow outside the stent cage but remain contained within the graft fabric, which reduces stress on the stent cage. This unique design may create the CT appearance of dye residing outside the stent (Fig. 7.40). Familiarity with this appearance will prevent mistakenly reporting an endoleak on post-EVAR surveillance imaging. In addition, since the

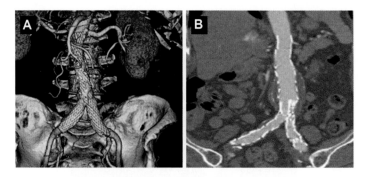

FIGURE 7.30. Illustration of the typical appearance of an AneuRx stent graft. Panel A is a volume-rendered image. Note the small diamond repetitive pattern which is typical for this stent graft. Panel B is a maximum intensity projection (MIP).

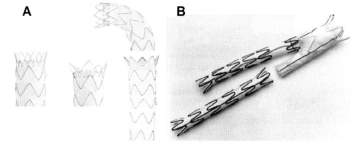

FIGURE 7.31. Illustration of two examples of a Talent suprarenal stent graft (World Medical/Medtronic, Sunrise, California). Panel A was adapted from Lin P, El Sayed H, Kougias P, et al. Endovascular repair of thoracic aortic disease: overview of current devices and clinical results. *Vascular*. 2007;15(4):179–190. Panel B was reproduced with kind permission from Springer. Copyright 2001. Dietrich E. AAA stent grafts: current developments. *J Invasive Cardiol*. 2001;13(5):1–13. This graft will appear to cross the renal arteries. To avoid the misdiagnosis of stent migration, a prior knowledge of the stent graft type will aid in evaluating a computed tomographic (CT) angiogram.

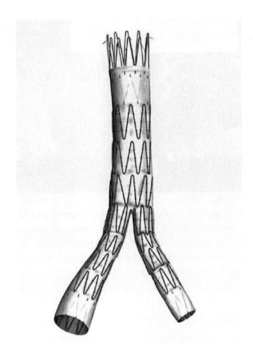

FIGURE 7.32. A Zenith endovascular stent graft (Cook, Bloomington, Indiana) (Reproduced with kind permission from Springer. Copyright 2001. Dietrich E. AAA stent grafts: current developments. *J Invasive Cardiol.* 2001;13(5):1–13).

Powerlink is not modular it is rarely associated with type III endoleaks. The CT appearance of this stent graft is that of large diamonds.

CT angiography should be the gold standard for pre-EVAR planning. Many measurements and assessments are necessary before EVAR is performed to determine if the patient is a candidate for EVAR (Figs. 7.41 and 7.42). First and foremost, the aneurysm must be accurately measured and characterized. The true maximum diameter and length of the aneurysm must be determined. Orthogonal off-axis views for true cross-sectional aneurysm area measurements are required to assure accuracy. Areas of layered thrombus should be

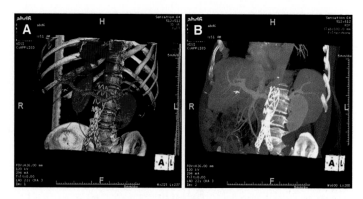

FIGURE 7.33. Panels A (volume-rendered image) and B (maximum intensity projection, MIP) illustrate the typical computed tomographic (CT) appearance of a Zenith stent (Cook, Bloomington, Indiana) and its typically visible large "zig zags." This modular stent extends from below the renal arteries to the aortic bifurcation and into the iliac arteries. It is deployed in modular sections.

included when measuring the maximum diameter of the aneurysm and should be noted to assure that the stent may be easily advanced. An accurate centerline measurement must also be made to quantify the length of aorta from the renal arteries to the bifurcation of the aorta and from renal arteries to hypogastric arteries. A centerline measurement is required to account for vessel tortuosity (Fig. 7.43).

Next, the aneurysm neck must be characterized (Figs. 7.41 and 7.42). The aortic diameter at the lowest renal artery and at the beginning of the aneurysm is measured. For proper stent apposition, these measurements may not differ by more than 10%. Accessory renal arteries should be noted. To accurately characterize the aneurysm neck, oblique views may be needed. A centerline measurement of neck length must also be acquired and the quality of the neck must be determined. It should be assessed for thrombus, calcium, shape, and angulation. Angulation in the anterior–posterior direction is more optimal for successful stenting than that in the lateral angulation. Figure 7.44 demonstrates various aneurysm neck characteristics.

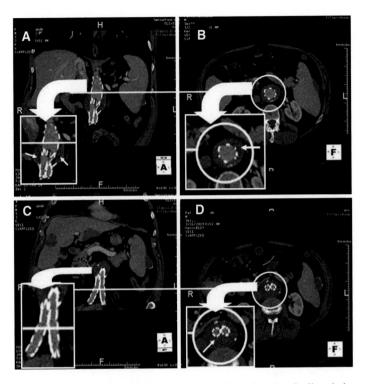

FIGURE 7.34. The Zenith stent (Cook, Bloomington, Indiana) in multiplanar reformat (MPR). Panels A and B are long axes and panels C and D are the corresponding axial images through the planes depicted by the *white line*. The thrombosed aneurysm outside the stent is visible in these MPR images (*straight white arrows*). The *small boxes* outlined in *white* are magnified views.

In addition, the centerline length of the iliac arteries from the aortic bifurcation to the hypogastric arteries is needed to determine the suitability of the iliac arteries for distal stent apposition (Fig. 7.41). The diameter and quality of the iliac vessels must also be determined. Procedural hindrances include iliac artery calcification and tortuosity. Since EVAR necessarily occludes the IMA, hypogastric artery patency must be assured to preserve the necessary

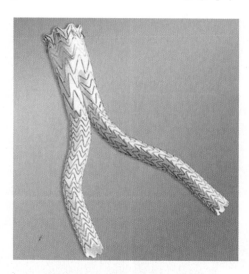

Figure 7.35. The Gore Excluder endovascular stent (W.L. Gore & Associates, Flagstaff, Arizona). Its "zig zags" appear smaller in a computed tomographic (CT) image than those of the Cook Zenith stent (Reprinted with kind permission from Anderson Publishing Ltd. Copyright 2005. Kinney TB, Rivera-Sanfeliz GM, Ferrara S. Stent grafts for abdominal and thoracic aortic disease. *Appl Radiol.* 2005;34:9–19).

collateral network to the viscera and prevent iatrogenic mesenteric ischemia.

Finally, the femoral artery must be assessed to determine if arterial access is suitable for the EVAR procedure. The femoral artery must be at least 7 mm (24 French) so that the procedural sheath may be accommodated within the artery.

After market programs such as the Medical Metrx Solutions (MMS) system automate the pre-EVAR planning process and allow the virtual fitting of stent grafts to assure that the stent grafts are appropriately sized and that the seal zones are adequate. These systems may also be used for post-EVAR surveillance using FEA to analyze post-EVAR aneurysm tension and volume. For the MMS system, 0.5-mm slice thickness CT images are necessary. Using advanced graphics workstations and

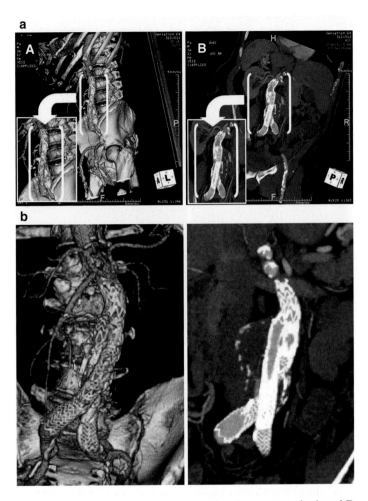

FIGURE 7.36. (a) Panels A (volume-rendered reconstruction) and B (maximum intensity projection, MIP) depict the typical computed tomographic (CT) appearance of the Gore Excluder endovascular stent graft (W.L. Gore & Associates, Flagstaff, Arizona). The smaller panels outlined in *white* are magnified images of the stent graft depicted in the main panels. (b) A magnified example of the Gore Excluder endovascular stent graft (W.L. Gore & Associates, Flagstaff, Arizona).

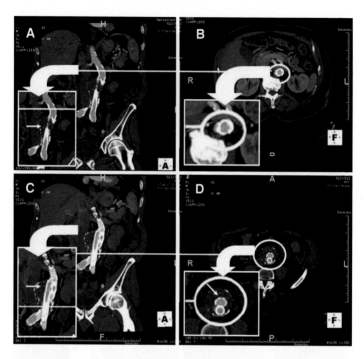

FIGURE 7.37. Demonstration of the cross-sectional appearance of the Gore Excluder (W.L. Gore & Associates, Flagstaff, Arizona) shown in Fig. 7.36 at the cross-sectional plane noted by the *white line*. The *small boxes* outlined in *white* are magnified images. The thrombosed aneurysm is again visible (*white arrows* in panels A, C and D).

proprietary software, MMS technicians create patient-specific three-dimensional computer models from two-dimensional CT scan data. Treatment planning software then offers detailed three-dimensional computer models combined with corresponding two-dimensional images and sophisticated quantification tools. This system is a powerful tool for patient selection, disease assessment, treatment planning, and surveillance.

The post-EVAR surveillance program is extensive and similar to the surveillance necessary after surgical repair. A follow-up CT angiogram is required at 1 month, 6 months, 12 months, and then annually for 5 years. If no complications

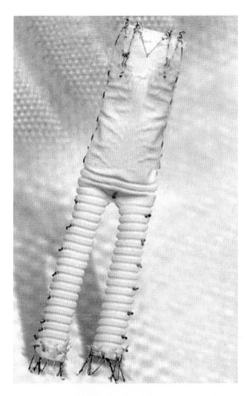

FIGURE 7.38. Depiction of an Ancure endovascular stent graft (Guidant, Menlo Park, California) (Reproduced with kind permission from Springer. Copyright 2001. Dietrich E. AAA stent grafts: current developments. *J Invasive Cardiol.* 2001;13(5):1–13).

or problems are noted, the post–5-year follow-up is individualized. For example, if the excluded lumen is shrinking, a surveillance CT angiogram may be considered every other year or a change to ultrasound surveillance may be considered.

Follow-up surveillance imaging studies are performed to identify the development of endoleaks, to assure that the excluded aneurysm sack is shrinking, to rule out kinks and fractures, and to identify stent migration. Delayed images are obtained to exclude subtle endoleaks. Volume calculations

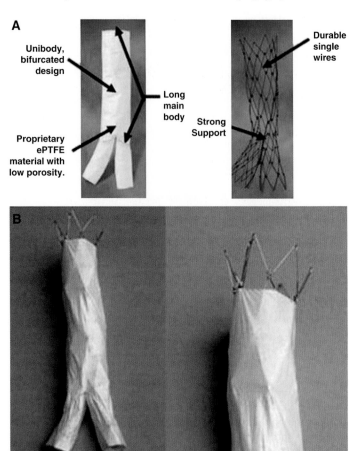

FIGURE 7.39. Illustration of the Endologix endovascular stent graft (Endologix, Irvine, California): Images in panel A were provided with kind permission from Endologix Inc. Lin P, El Sayed H, Kougias P, et al. Endovascular repair of thoracic aortic disease: overview of current devices and clinical results. *Vascular*. 2007;15(4):179–190. Panel B was reproduced with kind permission from Springer. Copyright 2001. Dietrich E. AAA stent grafts: current developments. *J Invasive Cardiol*. 2001;13(5):1–13).

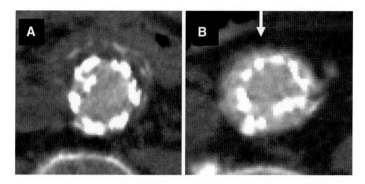

FIGURE 7.40. Panels A and B depict the typical appearance of the Endologix endovascular stent graft in a multiplanar reformatted (MPR) image. The graft material is only attached to the endoskeleton of the stent at the proximal (panel A) and distal ends. Thus at these points, no dye is seen outside the stent struts (panel A). However, between these attachment points in the body of the stent graft (panel B), the graft material floats freely away from the stent endoskeleton. Thus, dye is seen outside the stent struts but is contained within the graft material (panel B). Thus a distinct "circle" of dye is seen outside the stent struts but within the graft material. No dye is seen in the aneurysm itself (*white arrow* in panel B).

and diameter measurements are used to gauge the size of the excluded aneurysm. Because of concerns over contrast administration and radiation exposure, pressure sensors percutaneously placed inside the excluded aneurysm lumen at the time of the initial procedure have been developed (CardioMems™, Fig. 7.45). This device may be wise in patients with renal insufficiency where CT angiographic surveillance with contrast dye may not be ideal.

Endoleaks are classified into five types (Table 7.1 and Fig. 7.46). Type I is an attachment leak. Blood flow into the aneurysm sac originates from a seal zone caused by incompetent proximal or distal attachment sites. Type I leaks are prone to rupture and should be corrected promptly. Type II endoleaks represent retrograde flow into the aneurysm sac from a branch vessel or from collateral blood flow into the aneurysm. Possible culprit sources of a type II endoleak

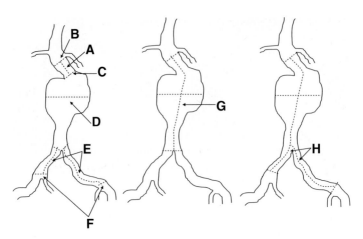

FIGURE 7.41. A cartoon demonstrating the necessary pre-endovascular aneurysm repair (EVAR) measurements. "A" is the length of the neck between the lowest renal artery and the beginning of the aneurysm. "B" is the width of the proximal neck, and "C" is the width of the distal neck. These two diameters may not differ by more than 10%. "D" is the true cross-sectional maximum aneurysm width (off-axis views may be necessary). "E" is the length of the iliac arteries to the point of origin of the hypogastric arteries. "F" is the diameter of the iliac arteries just proximal to the hypogastric arteries. "G" is the centerline length from the proximal neck to the aortic bifurcation. "H" is the centerline length from the proximal neck to the origin of the hypogastric arteries bilaterally.

include the IMA, the internal iliac artery, lumbar artery to hypogastric artery collaterals, or the arc of Riolan via the wandering artery of Drummond (most common). Type II endoleaks occur in up to 40% of patients undergoing EVAR.[161, 162] These endoleaks may often be corrected by selective therapeutic embolization of the culprit branch or collateral. It is reasonable to survey this type of leak for aneurysm sac enlargement prior to definitive therapy.

A Type III endoleak is a mid-graft defect or a defect in a modular connection site. Type III leaks have the same rupture potential as type I leaks and should also be repaired quickly.

Fabric porosity defines a type IV endoleak. The existence of type V leaks is debated. Here, it is proposed that heme extravasates through the graft material itself and into the

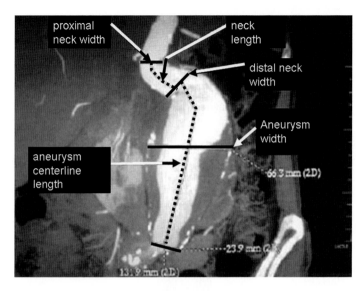

FIGURE 7.42. A "live" example of some of the necessary pre-endovascular aneurysm repair (EVAR) planning measurements.

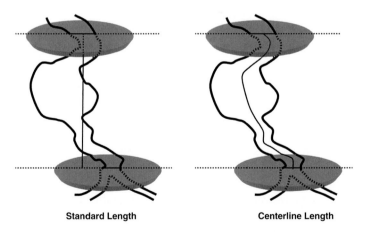

FIGURE 7.43. A cartoon depiction of the difference between a standard length measurement and a centerline length measurement. The standard measurement does not account for vessel tortuosity while the centerline measurement takes vessel tortuosity into account and should be used for all aneurysm length measurements.

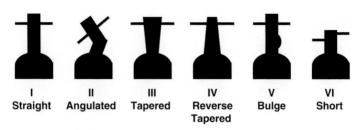

I	II	III	IV	V	VI
Straight	**Angulated**	**Tapered**	**Reverse Tapered**	**Bulge**	**Short**

FIGURE 7.44. A cartoon depicting various aneurysm neck characteristics.

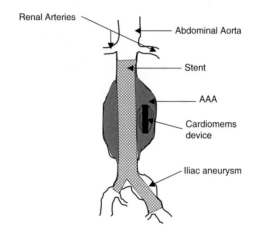

FIGURE 7.45. The CardioMems™ device which is placed percutaneously into the excluded aneurysm sac at the time of the endovascular aneurysm repair (EVAR) procedure. AAA: Abdominal aortic aneurysm.

aneurysm sac. The excluded aneurysm enlarges without evidence of an endoleak. The proposed cause of a type V endoleak is endotension where it is hypothesized that there is a pressure transmission through the thrombus at the stent attachment site or that there exists a low slow endoleak that is unidentifiable with standard imaging modalities.

Figures 7.47–7.51 depict patient examples of EVAR endoleaks. Figure 7.52 demonstrates the typical appearance of a surgically repaired AAA.

TABLE 7.1. Five types of endoleaks.

Type	Description	Characteristics
Type I	Attachment leak	– Usually seen at distal or proximal segment – Arises from inner edge of aneurysm sac
Type II	Branch or collateral flow	– Seen at distal or proximal stent segment – Arises from outer edge of aneurysm sec
Type III	Graft defect or modular disconnection	– Seen in middle of stent segment or at modular connection site – Arises from inner edge of aneurysm sac
Type IV	Fabric porosity	– More diffusely seen throughout the stent length – Arises from inner edge of aneurysm sac
Type V	Endotension	– Enlarging aneurysm sac with no visualized endoleak

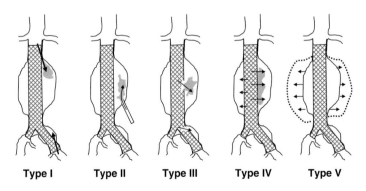

Type I   **Type II**   **Type III**   **Type IV**   **Type V**

FIGURE 7.46. Demonstration in cartoon format of the five endoleak classifications. Type I is an attachment leak. Type II is a leak from a collateral vessel. Type III is a modular leak or a graft defect. Type IV is a leak emanating from fabric porosity. Type V is an endotension leak.

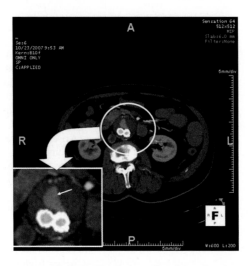

FIGURE 7.47. An endoleak. The *box* outlined in *white* is a magnification of the encircled area. The endoleak is denoted by the *small white arrow* in the magnified panel. The type of endoleak cannot be determined from this image alone but the fact that it arises from the inner half part of the aneurysmal sac suggests that it is either a type I or type III leak. A type IV leak would be more likely to be more diffuse in its appearance.

EVAR Versus Surgical AAA Repair

The major objective of AAA repair is to prevent rupture. There are no definite guidelines to help decide between EVAR and surgical repair. The method of repair is individualized to the patient. In general, EVAR is often the first choice unless the patient is not a candidate based on the pre-EVAR planning evaluation.

Open repair of AAA is considered major surgery with the potential for major complications, including death and paralysis. EVAR has been shown to reduce the need for blood transfusions, to shorten the acute hospital stay, and to decrease procedural-related mortality.[163, 164] Carpenter, however, reported that the initial procedural-related length of stay benefit with EVAR was lost during the first year of

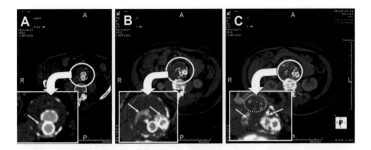

FIGURE 7.48. Demonstration of a type II endoleak (*small white arrows*). Analysis of multiple axial planes is necessary to make this determination. Panels A to C represent progressively more caudal axial planes. The *white boxes* are magnifications of the encircled areas. The endoleak(s) are denoted by the *white arrows* in the magnified panels. Panel A shows the endoleak emanating from the inner portion of the aneurysmal sac. However, as the planes progress caudally, the leak is seen to actually emanate from the outer portion of the sac defining a type II leak (panel C). In addition, panel C demonstrates other focal contrasted regions within the aneurysm sac (*dotted circle*), suggesting other collateral vessels emptying contrast into the excluded aneurysm sac.

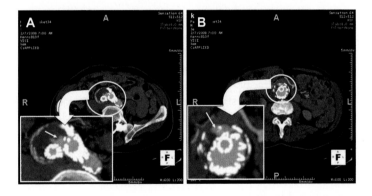

FIGURE 7.49. Demonstration of a probable modular leak (type III). Its location at the inner portion of the sac and in the region of a modular connection (panel A) suggests a type III endoleak. Panels A and B are axial images progressing superiorly. The *white boxes* are magnified images of the encircled areas. The *small white arrows* in the magnified panels point to the endoleak.

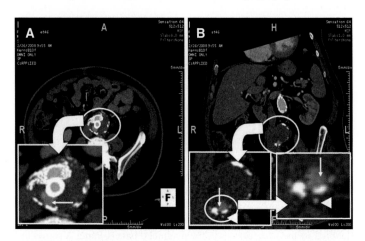

FIGURE 7.50. Illustration of a type II endoleak. Panels A and B progress superiorly. The *white boxes* in panels A and B are magnifications of the encircled areas. The endoleak is noted by the *small white arrows* in the magnified panels. Panel A does not permit classification of the endoleak. However, panel B shows that the endoleak emanates from the outer portion of the aneurysm sac and the *white arrowhead* points to the collateral vessel causing the leak.

follow-up due to readmissions for subsequent aneurysm-related procedures.[165] The total hospital stay did not differ at 12 months between the 2 groups.[166]

Reduced intraoperative mortality with EVAR has not been reported in all studies and improvement in long-term survival has not yet been demonstrated.[163, 164, 166, 167] However, in hospital mortality and 30-day mortality favors EVAR. Brewster[181] reported a 1.8% 30-day mortality after EVAR and a 97.6% and 94% 5-year and 9-year freedom from rupture, respectively.[167] In this study, an aneurysm-related death was avoided in 96.1%.

Predictors of aneurysm-related death were family history of aneurysmal disease, need for any reintervention, and renal artery disease.[168] Reintervention within 10 years was required in 10% (94% catheter-based).[168] Successful reintervention was reported on 84% of all reinterventions.[168] Predictors of reintervention

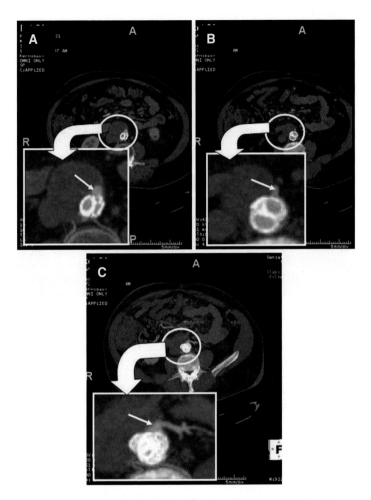

FIGURE 7.51. Another example of a type II endoleak. The figure format is similar to that of Figs. 7.47–7.50. The *small white arrows* in the insets show the endoleak. Panel C points to the collateral vessel entering the aneurysm sac.

were first-generation devices and late onset endoleaks. Later generation devices correlated with improved outcomes.[168] Cumulative freedom from conversion to open repair was 93% at

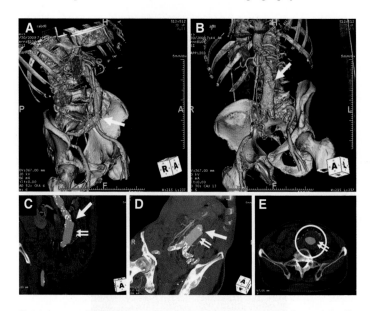

FIGURE 7.52. Illustration of the typical appearance of a surgically corrected abdominal aortic aneurysm (AAA). Panels A and B are volume-rendered reconstructions. Panels C and D are maximum intensity projections (MIP) in long-axis planes and panel E is axial plane MIP. Note the sharp angulation denoted by the *white arrow* in panel A. These types of angles are rarely seen in natural anatomy. Note the abrupt arterial diameter change denoted by the *thick white arrows* seen in panels B, C, and D. In addition, panels C and D highlight (*double white arrows*) the unnaturally smooth and straight appearance of the endograft. Finally, the *double arrow* in panel C points to the typically smooth axial outline within the excluded aneurysm sac typically seen with a surgically placed endograft.

5–9 years.[168] Cumulative survival was 52% at 5 years. Rupture following EVAR resulted from endograft failure or from failure to undergo post-EVAR surveillance.[168] Paralysis has been reported in 3% of EVAR procedures for thoracic aortic aneurysms and not reported in EVAR for AAA.[168] Most studies have shown a 4–5% operative mortality for surgery.[169-171]

Most recently, three interesting studies have been reported. Mani et al.[172] demonstrated improved long-term survival after elective abdominal aortic aneurysm repair between the two time periods from 1987 to 1999 and from 2000 to 2005. These data published in 2009 come from the Swedish Vascular Registry and demonstrate an increase in actuarial survival from 67.1% to 72.2% over these two periods. EVAR was offered starting in 2000 and was used 5.1% of the time between 2000 and 2005. Elective repair resulted in an 8.9-year survival on average while emergent repair of AAA ruptures allowed an average survival of 5 years. Relative long-term survival after elective repair was higher among men than women.

Another study by Veith et al.[173] published in 2009 analyzed the EVAR experience in treating ruptured AAA from 49 centers in Europe, Canada, and the United States. A total of 1,037 patients were treated with EVAR while 763 patients underwent open repair. The overall 30-day mortality in the EVAR group was 21%. EVAR was used in all patients where the anatomy permitted its use. The outcomes from 13 centers utilizing EVAR for AAA rupture were analyzed versus open repair for those with unsuitable anatomy. The 30-day mortality for EVAR was 19.7% versus 36% for open repair. While this was a retrospective study, a randomized trial called IMPROVE funded by the National Institute of Health Research in the United Kingdom is recruiting 600 patients with documented AAA rupture to be randomly assigned to open repair versus EVAR.

Finally, the OVER trial by Lederle et al.[174] demonstrated a lower risk of death in the first 30 days after EVAR compared with open surgical repair for AAA. In this trial, 881 Veteran Affairs patients (mean age 70 years) were randomly assigned to EVAR versus surgery. Only 0.5% of the patients in the EVAR group died in the first 30 days compared to 3% in the surgery group. No statistical difference in mortality at 2 years between the groups was noted.

Physicians must openly inform their patients, if possible, of the risks associated with EVAR including endoleaks (occurring in 25% of the EVAR group in the OVER study), the potential need for secondary therapeutic procedures (needed in 18 of 110 endoleak patients in the OVER study), and the substantial radiation and dye exposure experienced by EVAR patients both acutely during the procedure and with surveillance CT angiograms.

7.2.4.2 Common Iliac Arteries

Isolated common iliac artery aneurysms without AAA are rare. One-third to one-half of common iliac artery aneurysms are bilateral. Most are asymptomatic at the time of discovery. Rupture usually occurs at ≥3 cm and thus corrective procedures should be considered when common iliac aneurysms reach this size.[175,176] While most aneurysms are atherosclerotic in nature, aneurysms may occur in association with various illnesses such as Ehlers–Danlos syndrome (Fig. 7.53).

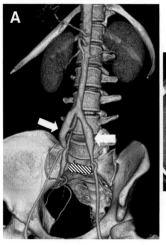
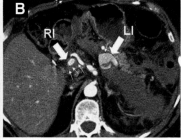

FIGURE 7.53. Panels A and B depict bilateral iliac artery aneurysms in two different patients with Ehlers–Danlos syndrome. Panel A is a volume-rendered, segmented reconstruction demonstrating involvement of the iliac arteries (*white arrows*) and the right hypogastric artery (*black and white striped arrow*). Panel B is an axial multiplanar reformat (MPR) showing a left iliac artery (LI) aneurysm (*thick white arrow*) with a small amount of thrombus (*thin white arrow*) and severely thrombosed right iliac artery (RI) aneurysm (*three thin white arrows*) with a narrowed lumen (Reproduced with kind permission from the American Roentgen Ray Society. Copyright 2007. Zilocchi M, Macedo T, Oderich G, et al. Vascular Ehlers-Danlos syndrome: imaging findings. *Am J Roentgenol.* 2007;189:712–717).

7.2.4.3 Visceral Arteries

Visceral artery aneurysms may be insidious because they are often asymptomatic and difficult to diagnose unless incidentally discovered on an imaging study. Some studies have reported that with the exception of renal artery aneurysms (which rarely rupture), 50% of all visceral artery aneurysms present with rupture.[177] The mortality observed with surgical repair of ruptured visceral artery aneurysms is over 25%.[177]

Splenic and Hepatic Arteries

Splenic and hepatic artery aneurysms are rare but potentially fatal, most often due to rupture. They comprise 80% of all visceral artery aneurysms. The reported incidence of splenic artery aneurysms ranges from 0.05% up to 10% and represent the most common form of visceral artery aneurysm.[178-180] Figures 7.54 and 7.55 demonstrate examples of splenic artery aneurysms.

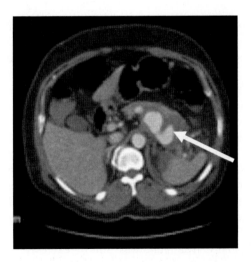

FIGURE 7.54. An example of a large splenic artery aneurysm (*white arrow*). Splenic and hepatic artery aneurysms may be overlooked if the splenic and hepatic arteries are not routinely evaluated in, along their entire length.

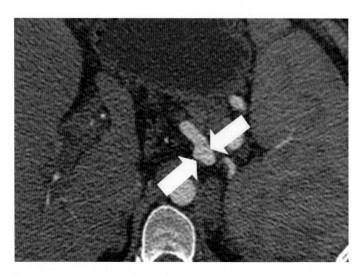

FIGURE 7.55. An example of a more subtle splenic artery aneurysm (between the *white arrows*).

Atherosclerosis is the most important single pathophysiologic cause of splenic and hepatic artery aneurysms. Congenital defects have also been implicated. These arteries are noted to have an abrupt absence of the internal elastic lamina and media. This abnormality may lead to spontaneous rupture without aneurysm formation. Trauma may also induce rupture. Mycotic aneurysms have been documented.[178]

These aneurysms are usually asymptomatic unless rupture occurs or unless they grow to a size that affects surrounding structures.[181] While pregnancy does not cause splenic or hepatic artery aneurysms, it is a factor that induces rupture, and rupture is more prevalent during pregnancy. Therefore, these aneurysms should be corrected if pregnancy is planned.[182]

Traditionally, treatment was almost exclusively surgical. However, endovascular stenting has been reported. Since rupture is often fatal, repair is recommended if symptoms are present or for aneurysms >2 cm. All pseudoaneurysms should be repaired.

Isolated hepatic artery aneurysms are rare. Repair is recommended if concomitant FMD is present, or if >2 cm, or if concomitant polyarteritis nodosa. In addition, hepatic artery aneurysms should be repaired if liver transplantation is planned.

Mesenteric Arteries

Mesenteric artery aneurysms are even less common than splenic or hepatic artery aneurysms, representing only 6–7% of all visceral artery aneurysms.[179, 183] Celiac artery and SMA aneurysms are also prone to rupture at sizes ≥2 cm. Elective repair should thus be considered for size ≥2 cm.[184] Men and those with noncalcified aneurysms have the highest risk of rupture. In one study, no rupture was observed in those taking beta-blockers.[183] The operative mortality for ruptured aneurysms was 38% and no deaths were noted in elective repairs.[183] Figure 7.56 is an example of an SMA aneurysm.

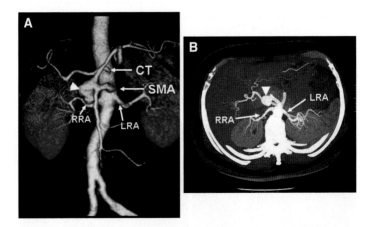

FIGURE 7.56. Depiction of a large superior mesenteric artery (SMA) aneurysm (*white arrowhead*). Panel A is a volume-rendered, segmented reconstruction. CT: Celiac trunk. RRA: Right renal artery. LRA: Left renal artery (Reprinted with kind permission from 3D Diagnostix Inc (www.3ddx.com). Copyright 2007. Image available at www.3ddx.com/cv_sample6.html).

7.2.5 Renal Artery Disease

7.2.5.1 Renal Artery Aneurysms

Renal artery aneurysms are rare and occur in less than 0.5% of the population. Fibrodysplasia is the most prevalent finding associated with renal artery aneurysms, while atherosclerosis is a rare cause. Rupture is unlikely in most patients but is more common in women of reproductive age and during pregnancy.[198] Bilateral renal artery aneurysms are present 20% of the time,[198] while multiple unilateral renal artery aneurysms are noted in 30% of patients.[198] Surgical treatment should be considered for aneurysms 1.5–2 cm and is mandatory for all aneurysms >2 cm or for patients with symptoms of flank pain (which may, however, be coincidental).[198] Of largest concern are non-calcified aneurysms ≥2 cm because of an increased rupture risk particularly during pregnancy.[199, 200] Endovascular stenting with exclusion of a renal artery aneurysm has been reported. In rare cases, renal artery aneurysms may be embolized. Figure 7.57 depicts an example of a right renal artery aneurysm.

7.2.5.2 Renal Artery Atherosclerosis

Atherosclerosis accounts for 90% of all cases of renal artery stenosis (RAS). Most of the remaining 10% of RAS are

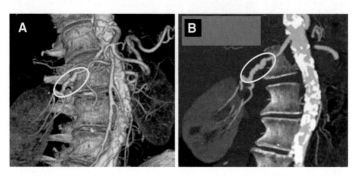

FIGURE 7.57. An example of a right renal artery aneurysm. Panel A is a volume-rendered image while panel B is a thick maximum intensity projection (MIP). The aneurysm is circled in *white* in both panels A and B. The aorta is highly calcified.

caused by fibromuscular dysplasia (FMD) and vasculitis. Other rare causes include thrombosed renal artery aneurysms. Since renal artery atherosclerosis is an extension of abdominal aortic atherosclerosis, renal artery stenoses are often located at the ostium and proximal segments of the artery. Significant RAS is defined as a ≥50% stenosis. Hemodynamically significant stenoses are those ≥75%.

The overall prevalence of RAS in patients ≥65 years is nearly 7%. In this age group, RAS is seen in 5.5% of women, 9.1% of men, 6.9% of whites, and 6.7% of blacks.[201] High-risk populations include patients undergoing screening renal arteriogram at the time of invasive coronary angiography where RAS is noted in nearly 30% of patients.[202, 203] In patients with peripheral arterial disease (PAD) the prevalence of RAS is as high as 22–59%.[204, 205] A very high prevalence of carotid artery disease is noted in patients with significant RAS and thus, if significant RAS is diagnosed, a carotid sonogram should be performed.[206] More severe kidney dysfunction, more advanced hypertension and coexisting cardiovascular disease predict poorer outcomes in patients with RAS.[207] Furthermore, the presence of asymptomatic RAS is a powerful predictor of mortality.[208]

Atherosclerotic RAS is a progressive disease. Treatment for atherosclerotic RAS includes medical management, angioplasty without stenting, angioplasty with stenting, and surgery. The goals of treatment include improvement in uncontrolled hypertension, maintenance of, or improvement in, kidney function, and perhaps improvement in quality of life. The mainstay for revascularization therapy is angioplasty with stenting. Surgical revascularization is usually reserved for complicated renal artery anatomy or concomitant perirenal artery abdominal aneurysm repair.[207]

Overall, the evidence does not indicate superiority of either percutaneous or surgical treatment for RAS.[207] Mortality outcomes, renal function, and blood pressure management seem to be similar in both groups.[207] Restenosis rates after stenting range from 10% to 21%.[207] No difference in quality of life has been demonstrated among any of the treatment options.[207]

Further study is required to answer the important questions regarding RAS treatment. The CORAL trial is underway and will compare medical management versus renal artery stenting for RAS. This trial is enrolling patients with RAS ≥60%, who suffer from systolic hypertension while on two or more antihypertensive medications. Those with advanced chronic kidney disease (serum creatinine >3.0 mg/dL), atrophic kidneys (<7 cm), or those with significant concomitant cardiovascular disease are excluded.

Figures 7.58 and 7.59 are examples of renal artery atherosclerotic disease. Figures 7.60–7.62 are examples of renal artery stents.

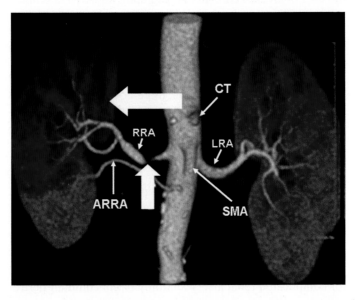

FIGURE 7.58. A volume-rendered image demonstrating a severe stenosis of the right renal artery (*vertical block arrow*) resulting in hypoperfusion of the majority of the right kidney (*horizontal block arrow*). RRA: Right renal artery. LRA: Left renal artery. The accessory right renal artery (ARRA) is normally perfusing a small portion of the right lower kidney. CT: Celiac trunk. SMA: Superior mesenteric artery (Reproduced with kind permission from the American Roentgen Ray Society. Copyright 2007. Parrish F. Volume CT: state-of-the-art reporting. *Am J Roentgenol.* 2007;189:528–534).

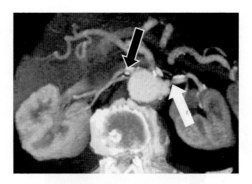

FIGURE 7.59. A maximum intensity projection (MIP) demonstrating mild calcific atherosclerotic disease of the ostium of the right renal artery (*black arrow*). The left renal artery has a tight proximal stenosis (*white arrow*). The left kidney is atrophic.

7.2.5.3 Fibromuscular Dysplasia of the Renal Arteries

Fibromuscular dysplasia (FMD) is a noninflammatory, nonatherosclerotic disorder that leads to arterial stenoses. It may affect nearly every arterial bed, but most commonly involves the renal arteries (60–75%)[209] and the internal carotid arteries (25–30%).[209] Approximately 25% of patients have multiple involved arterial beds.[209] Clinical manifestations vary depending on the affected arterial bed. The most frequent presentations include hypertension, transient ischemic attack, and stroke.

FMD is two to ten times more common in adult females than in adult males but no gender prevalence is noted in children.[211] FMD is most often diagnosed in patients younger than 50 years of age. The most notable exception is FMD of the cerebral circulation where the mean age at diagnosis is 62 years.[210, 212]

Visceral arterial FMD is a rare finding. If present, the celiac, SMA, IMA, hepatic, and splenic arteries are most often involved. The iliac, femoral, popliteal, and peroneal arteries may also be affected.[213,214] The subclavian arteries are the most commonly involved upper extremity arteries though brachial and axillary arterial involvement have been reported.[215]

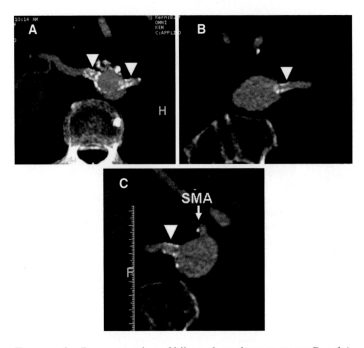

FIGURE 7.60. Demonstration of bilateral renal artery stents. Panel A is a maximum intensity projection (MIP) of both stents (*arrowheads*), and the stent lumen cannot be seen. Panels B (left renal artery) and C (right renal artery) are multiplanar reformats (MPR). In these images the stent lumen can be clearly seen and both stents are patent, without significant in-stent stenoses (panels B and C, *arrowheads*). SMA: Superior mesenteric artery. Using the MPR is one method to evaluate the stent lumen.

FMD is categorized into five types depending on the affected arterial layer and the pathologic composition (Table 7.2).[216] Medial fibroplasia is most common (75–80%) and demonstrates the classic "string of beads" appearance caused by alternating segments of fibromuscular constrictions and aneurysmal dilation. The aneurysmal areas are characterized by the absence of the internal elastic lamina. Total occlusion is uncommon.[217]

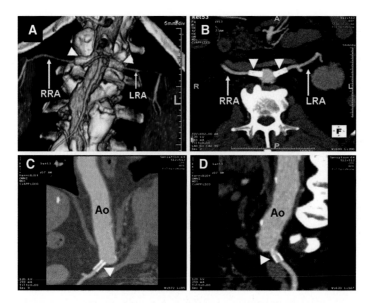

FIGURE 7.61. Panel A is a volume-rendered image demonstrating the presence of bilateral renal artery stents (*white arrowheads*). Panel B is a maximum intensity projection (MIP) illustrating both stents but the lumen cannot be evaluated using MIP. Panels C (right renal artery) and D (left renal artery) are curved multiplanar reformats (cMPR) and demonstrate the stent lumen nicely (*white arrowheads*). cMPR is another method with which to evaluate the stent lumen. RRA: Right renal artery. LRA: Left renal artery. Ao: Aorta.

Intimal fibroplasia represents nearly 10% of FMD cases and results from circumferential or eccentric deposition of collagen into the intima. The internal elastic lamina may be intact, fragmented, or duplicated. There is no inflammatory or lipid component.

Perimedial fibroplasia demonstrates replacement of large parts of the media with collagen, causing an irregular thickening of the media. Total occlusion may occur with the development of collateral vasculature. In this type of FMD, the "bead" appearance is present in smaller sizes and in lesser numbers since aneurysm formation is uncommon.

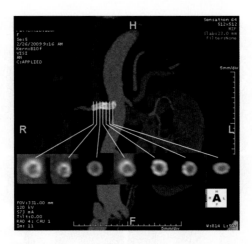

FIGURE 7.62. Depiction of multiple axial planes cutting through a left renal artery stent demonstrating stent patency.

Medial hyperplasia (1–2%) is a result of smooth muscle cell hyperplasia. Fibrosis is not seen.

Periarterial hyperplasia is rare (<1%). This type of FMD is caused by expansion of the fibrous adventitia where collagen extends into the periarterial fat. There is accompanying inflammation. This type may be associated with idiopathic retroperitoneal fibrosis.

The etiology of FMD is unknown. Genetic predisposition is noted since there is a reported familial occurrence.[215] Hormonal factors are also implicated since FMD is predominantly found in women of child-bearing age. Mechanical factors such as stretching of smooth muscle cells and trauma to the blood vessel wall as well as ischemia of the blood vessel wall due to fibrotic occlusion of the vasa vasorum have also been proposed.

Disease manifestations may result from ischemia, dissection, occlusion, aneurysm rupture, and embolization.[219, 220] Hypertension is the most common manifestation of renal artery FMD and is caused by activation of the renin-angiotensin system resulting from decreased renal perfusion. Progressive worsening of kidney function is rare.

TABLE 7.2. A pathological classification system for fibromuscular dysplasia (FMD).

Classification	Frequency	Pathology	Angiographic appearance
Medial dysplasia			
Medial fibroplasia	75–80%	Alternating areas of thinned media and thickened fibromuscular ridges containing collagen. Internal elastic lamina lost in some areas	String of beads appearance where the diameter of beading is larger than the diameter of artery
Perimedial fibroplasia	10–15%	Extensive collagen deposition in outer half of media	Beading where beads are smaller than the diameter of the artery
Medial hyperplasia	1–2%	True smooth muscle cell hyperplasia without fibrosis	Concentric smooth stenosis
Intimal fibroplasia			
	<10%	Circumferential or eccentric deposition of collagen in the intima. No lipid of inflammation component. Internal elastic lamina is fragmented or duplicated	Concentric focal band. Long smooth narrowing
Adventitial (periarterial) fibroplasia			
	<1%	Dense collagen replaces the fibrous tissue of the adventitia. May extend to the surrounding tissue	Sharply localized, tubular areas of stenosis

Cerebral artery FMD most commonly causes headache. Tinnitus, lightheadedness, amaurosis fugax, Horner's syndrome, transient ischemic attacks, and stroke may also occur.[210, 221] Carotid bruits may be absent.[222]

Lower extremity FMD may result in intermittent claudication, critical limb ischemia, or microembolism, causing painful, cyanotic toes.[214] Iliac dissection and rupture may rarely occur.[223] In the upper extremities, FMD may present as weakness, paresthesias, or upper extremity claudication.[215]

Rarely, chronic mesenteric ischemia, or intestinal angina, may result when two of the splanchnic arteries are occluded with a concomitant severe stenosis in the third. Infrequently, acute intestinal ischemia may be seen.

Renal artery dysplasia should be suspected in women under 50 years of age who demonstrate severe or refractory hypertension, in patients with the onset of hypertension before the age of 30 years, in patients who experience a sudden rise in blood pressure over a previously stable baseline, in those with a marked rise in the serum creatinine occurring after beginning an angiotensin converting enzyme inhibitor or angiotensin receptor blocker, or in patients with an epigastric bruit.

Digital subtraction angiography (DSA) is the gold standard for the diagnosis of FMD.[213] Medial fibroplasia will appear as a "string of beads." In this case, the diameter of the beads is larger than the arterial diameter. When the beads are less numerous and smaller than the diameter of the artery itself, perimedial fibroplasia is usually the pathologic diagnosis. Medial hyperplasia and intimal fibroplasia demonstrate concentric smooth stenoses whereas periarterial fibroplasia demonstrates sharply localized tubular stenoses. Several noninvasive imaging modalities may also be used to evaluate renal artery FMD including duplex ultrasound, CT angiography, and magnetic resonance angiography (MRA).[224-228] Figures 7.63 and 7.64 are examples of segmented volume-rendered CT angiograms demonstrating FMD of the renal arteries.

The conditions that most commonly mimic the presentation of FMD are atherosclerotic vascular disease and vasculitis. Patients with atherosclerosis are usually older and have typical

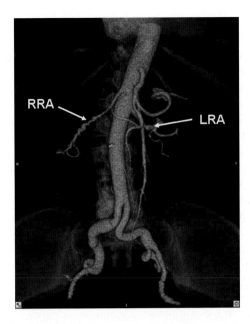

FIGURE 7.63. Depiction of a segmented volume-rendered image demonstrating fibromuscular dysplasia (FMD) of the renal arteries. Note the "string of beads" appearance. RRA: Right renal artery. LRA: Left renal artery.

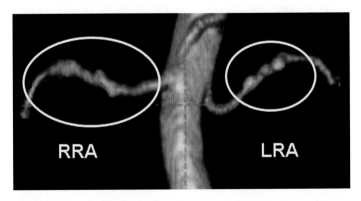

FIGURE 7.64. Another example of the classic "string of beads" appearance of fibromuscular dysplasia (FMD) (*circled regions*). RRA: Right renal artery. LRA: Left renal artery.

cardiovascular risk factors.[213] Older age, however, does not exclude the diagnosis of FMD. Other differentiating features between renal artery atherosclerosis and FMD are that atherosclerosis usually affects the ostium or proximal segments of the renal arteries whereas FMD most often involves the middle or distal segments. The "string of beads" appearance is only seen with FMD. While multiple systems are often involved with FMD and with vasculitis, patients with FMD lack the systemic symptoms experienced by vasculitis patients.

Invasive treatment for FMD with balloon angioplasty alone is usually effective. Patients who are treated medically should have blood pressures taken and serum creatinine measured every 3 months. Noninvasive imaging should be undertaken every 6–12 months. Progression is defined as new focal lesions, worsened stenosis, or enlargement of an aneurysm.[229, 230]

7.2.5.4 Screening for Renal Artery Stenosis

Screen for RAS should be undertaken as part of a work-up for secondary hypertension. Clinical clues suggesting RAS are age of hypertension onset <30 years or >55 years, abrupt onset hypertension, acceleration of hypertension, hypertension refractory to three or more medications, malignant hypertension, tobacco abuse, and abdominal bruit. Flash pulmonary edema, asymmetric kidney size and acute kidney failure, or hyperkalemia with angiotensin converting enzyme inhibitors or angiotensin receptor blocker initiation should also prompt a search for RAS.[177]

In addition, patients should be screened for RAS prior to starting hemodialysis or as part of the pretransplant evaluation. Surveillance post endovascular therapy is recommended at 6 months, 12 months, and then annually.[177]

7.3 Accuracy of Abdominal CT Angiography

Qanadili et al.[231] demonstrated that CT angiographic evaluation of AAA correlated well with surgical findings. Accessory renal arteries were accurately identified and the sensitivity and specificity of identifying stenoses of the celiac artery and SMA were both 100%. Other studies have shown CT angiography to have a 93% sensitivity, a 95% specificity, a 90% positive predictive value (PPV), and a 97% negative predictive value (NPV) for the characterization of the abdominal aorta.[231] The overall diagnostic accuracy for CT angiography for this indication was 94% in this study.[231] For abdominal aortic dissection, the sensitivity and specificity of CT angiography are both >99%.[231]

In addition, CT has been reported to have a sensitivity of 90% for the diagnosis of mesenteric ischemia.[234] New generations of multidetector row CT scanners have been shown to characterize the mesenteric vessels down to the smallest branches with excellent confirmation by DSA.[235] For inflammatory changes of the aorta, the sensitivity, specificity, and overall accuracy of CT angiography have been shown to be 83%, 100%, and 94%, respectively.[232, 233]

CT angiography is also the initial imaging test of choice for postendovascular AAA repair surveillance. In one study of post-EVAR surveillance, while CT angiography occasionally misclassified the type of endoleak, it correctly identified the presence of 95% of all endoleaks.[236] There has been shown to be an 86% agreement between CT angiography and DSA for endoleak recognition.[237] Axial multiplanar reformatting (MPR) is the most accurate reconstruction technique to identify the presence of an endoleak.[238]

The sensitivity and specificity of CT angiography for detecting and quantifying RAS are 96% and 99%, respectively.[239] The overall accuracy of CT angiography in detecting and quantifying RAS is reported to be in the 94% range.[240] In one RAS imaging study, the sensitivity, specificity, accuracy, PPV, and NPV of CT angiography were 100%, 98.6%, 96.9%, 97.6%, and 100%, respectively.[241]

CT angiography has variable sensitivity in detecting FMD.[225] However, the increased spatial resolution of 64 slice and greater CT machines will likely offer improved sensitivity in detecting FMD by offering more rapid image acquisition, thinner slices, three-dimensional volume rendering, diminished helical artifacts, and smaller contrast requirements. The choice of test should be based on local expertise.

7.4 Approach to Reading Abdominal Aortic CT Angiography

As with all diagnostic imaging, a systematic approach to reading an abdominal CT angiogram is necessary to assure accurate and complete evaluations. Readings should also focus on the clinical question at hand in order to provide clinical meaning to the study.

An anatomical overview is obtained using the three-dimensional volume-rendered reconstructions. Aneurysms are identified, clues to dissections and stenoses may be obtained, and peripheral arterial bypass grafts may be visualized, if present. Furthermore, endovascular stent grafts may be identified and clues to the presence of stent fractures, stent migration, or endoleaks may be seen.

Following the three-dimensional overview, maximum intensity projections (MIP) in multiple planes may be assessed to gain a more specific anatomical insight and to further identify problem areas. However, multiplanar reformatted (MPR) images are most often used to hone in on an arterial segment for a specific and complete analysis and for making a definitive diagnosis.

Calcified and noncalcified atherosclerosis should be qualitatively described and stenoses must be quantified. Each major aortic branch is identified and assessed including the celiac artery, SMA, renal arteries, and IMA. Lateral views are best for the celiac artery, SMA, and IMA (Fig. 7.65). Be sure to follow the hepatic and splenic arteries to their termination to identify occult aneurysms which are often asymptomatic and easily overlooked. These arteries may be tortuous. We have found that axial MPR analysis is the simplest and most effective method to assess the hepatic and splenic arteries. In addition, spinal branches may be assessed if clinically relevant.

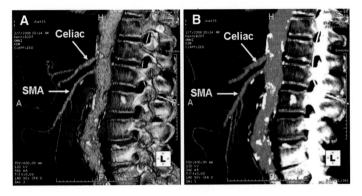

FIGURE 7.65. Demonstration of the utility of the lateral projections for identifying and evaluating the mesenteric vessels, especially the origin and proximal regions. Panel A is a volume-rendered reconstruction while panel B is a maximum intensity projection (MIP). Celiac: Celiac artery. SMA: Superior mesenteric artery.

Aneurysms are characterized, quantified and appropriate measurements are made, particularly if EVAR is being considered. In addition, the appropriate pre-EVAR planning measurements and characterizations are performed. Characterizing the location of the renal arteries is necessary. Identification of any accessory renal arteries is critical. If reading a post-EVAR study, assessments are made for graft fracture, migration, and for the presence and classification of endoleaks. Axial MPR is most accurate at identifying and classifying endoleaks.[238] In addition, measurements of the volume and size of the excluded aneurysm must be performed and documented.

It should be noted that surgical repair of an AAA is often performed by wrapping the native aorta around the graft to avoid aortoenteric fistula formation. Therefore, thrombus may be present around the graft. If there has been a surgical AAA repair, a thorough assessment of the body of the graft and of the graft anastomoses must be performed.

Reporting should be organized, concise, and clinically pertinent.

Chapter 8
Peripheral Arterial CT Angiography

8.1 Anatomy

The lower extremity peripheral arterial anatomy is represented in **Figs. 8.1 and 8.2.** The distal aorta bifurcates
into the common iliac arteries (CIA). The CIAs bifurcate

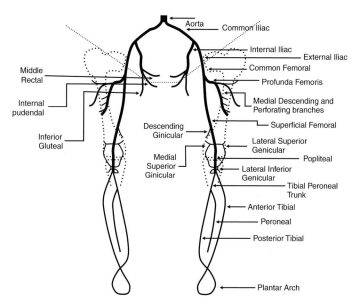

FIGURE 8.1. A cartoon depicting the normal peripheral arterial
anatomy beginning at the aorto-iliac bifurcation.

R. Pelberg, W. Mazur, *Vascular CT Angiography Manual*,   255
DOI: 10.1007/978-1-84996-260-5_8,
© Springer-Verlag London Limited 2011

FIGURE 8.2. Demonstration of the normal peripheral arterial anatomy in the axial plane. Panels A through L progress through the arterial tree beginning just before the aorto-iliac bifurcation (Panel A) and ending at the trifurcation into the three run-off vessels of the leg. Panel A demonstrates the aorta just before its bifurcation into the iliac vessels. The iliac vessels just after the bifurcation are seen in panel B and the more distal common iliac arteries are depicted in panel C. Panel D shows the external and internal iliac arteries just after their bifurcation and panel E demonstrates these arteries in a more caudal plane. Panel F shows the common femoral vessels, which are a continuation of the external iliac arteries just after the inguinal ligament. Panel G demonstrates the superficial femoral arteries and the profunda arteries just after their bifurcation from the common femoral vessels. Panel H shows the continuation of the superficial femoral and profunda arteries. Panel I depicts the popliteal arteries behind the knee, which are a continuation of the superficial femoral arteries. Panel J shows the bifurcation of the popliteal arteries into the anterior tibial arteries and the tibioperoneal trunks. Panel K shows the anterior tibial arteries as well as the peroneal and posterior tibial arteries after their bifurcation from the tibioperoneal trunk. These three run-off vessels continue to the ankle where the peroneal artery (coursing centrally down the midline of the leg) comes to an end in the distal calf and the anterior and posterior tibial arteries form the plantar arch. Panel L is a volume rendered reconstruction of the three run-off leg vessels and their anatomic relations. *Ao* Aorta, *RCI* right common iliac artery, *LCI* left common iliac artery, *REI*, right external iliac artery, *LEI* left external iliac artery, *RII*, right internal iliac artery, *LII* left internal iliac artery, *RCF* right common femoral artery, *LCF* left common femoral artery, *RSF* right superficial femoral artery, *LSF* left superficial femoral artery, *RPr* right profunda artery, *LPr* left profunda artery, *RPop* right popliteal artery, *LPop* left popliteal artery, *RAT* right anterior tibial artery. *LAT* left anterior tibial artery, *RTPT* right tibioperoneal trunk, *LTPT* left tibioperoneal trunk, *RPT* right posterior tibial artery, *LPT* left posterior tibial artery, *RP* right peroneal artery, *LP* left peroneal artery, *Pop* popliteal artery, *AT* anterior tibial artery, *TPT* tibioperoneal trunk, *PT* posterior tibial artery, *P* peroneal artery.

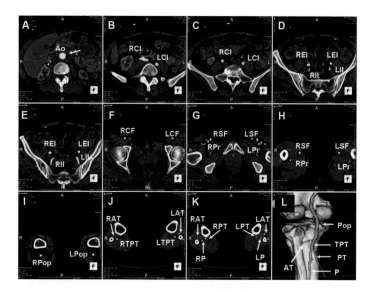

into the internal iliac artery and the external iliac artery, which then become the common femoral artery (CFA). The CIAs usually course anterior to the iliopsoas muscle but may run posterior to it. This normal variant should be noted.

Prior to becoming the superficial femoral artery (SFA), the CFA gives rise to the pudendal artery. The CFA becomes the SFA after giving rise to the obturator and the inferior epigastric arteries (usually, near the inguinal ligament). The SFA becomes the popliteal artery after the adductor canal, which is just above the knee.

The adductor canal (Hunter's canal) (Fig. 8.3) is an aponeurotic (membranes separating muscles) tunnel in the middle third of the thigh extending from the apex of the femoral triangle to the opening in the adductor magnus (adductor hiatus). The adductor canal courses between the anterior and medial thigh compartments. Its boundaries include the vastus medialis muscle (front and lateral) and the adductor longus and magnus muscles (posterior). It is covered by a strong

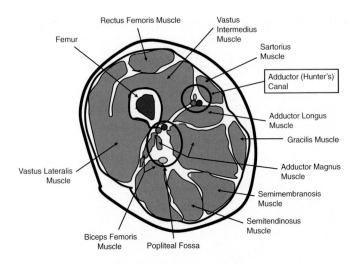

FIGURE 8.3. A cartoon depicting the adductor (Hunter's) canal (circled) through which the femoral vessels and nerves course. The popliteal fossa is also depicted. The yellow ovals represent nerves, the blue circles are veins and the red circles are arteries.

aponeurosis that extends from the vastus medialis muscle across the femoral vessels to the adductor longus and magnus muscles. Lying on the aponeurosis is the sartorius muscle. The adductor canal contains the femoral artery, femoral vein, and branches of the femoral nerve (specifically, the saphenous nerve, and the nerve to the vastus medialis).[242]

The popliteal artery bifurcates into the anterior tibial artery, which runs anteriorly and laterally and the tibial–peroneal trunk, which runs medially. The tibial–peroneal trunk splits to become the posterior tibial artery and the peroneal artery. The peroneal artery runs deep and usually in the midline, between the anterior and posterior tibial arteries. The posterior tibial artery courses medially. The anterior and posterior tibial arteries form the plantar arch.

The inflow vessels describe the abdominal aorta and the common and external iliac arteries and the femoral arteries. The outflow vessels include the popliteal, tibial, and peroneal arteries.

8.2 Disease Processes

8.2.1 Peripheral Arterial Atherosclerosis

The vast majority of patients with peripheral arterial disease (PAD) suffer from peripheral atherosclerosis. Other causes of PAD include aneurysms, fibromuscular dysplasia (FMD), thromboembolic disease, vasculitis, trauma, congenital abnormalities, and entrapment syndromes. In addition, arterial kinking, especially of the iliac artery, may result in endofibrosis and claudication. This entity is seen in endurance athletes such as cyclists. Other conditions that mimic PAD are deep venous thrombosis, musculoskeletal disorders, osteoarthritis, peripheral neuropathy, and spinal stenosis.

Atherosclerotic PAD is a common entity and affects large proportions of many worldwide populations. The total disease prevalence documented in several epidemiologic studies is between 3% and 10%.[243, 244, 245] Its prevalence increases to 15–20% in patients over 70 years.[243, 244, 245] Over eight million Americans suffer from PAD.[243] Using the ankle-brachial index (ABI) as a screen to detect asymptomatic PAD, the overall prevalence has been estimated at nearly 30%.[246] Similar to asymptomatic PAD, symptomatic PAD increases with age as well. Claudication is present in 3–6% of patients 40–60 years of age[247] and increases to 12–20% of those >65 years.[248]

Major risk factors implicated in the development of atherosclerotic PAD are diabetes, cigarette smoking, hypertension, and hyperlipidemia.[249, 250] While PAD is 1.5 times more prevalent in smokers,[251] diabetes is one of the strongest predictors for the development of PAD (twofold more prevalent).[252] For every 1% increase in hemoglobin A1c there is a 26% increased risk of PAD.[252] Furthermore, diabetics experience a 15% lifetime risk of developing a foot ulcer and 14–24% of diabetics with foot ulcers will eventually require an amputation.[253] Close to 85% of amputations may be prevented by early detection and appropriate treatment.[253] It is also known that diabetics suffer from more severe arterial disease and from poorer outcomes.[254]

The associations of hypertension and hyperlipidemia with PAD are much weaker than that for smokers and diabetics.[253] The most powerful lipid markers associated with PAD are triglycerides, HDL, and lipoprotein "a" (LPa). There is evidence that treatment of hyperlipidemia reduces both the progression of PAD and the incidence of intermittent claudication. Renal artery disease is also linked to PAD.[253] Nonwhite ethnicity is also a risk factor. African-American ethnicity increases the risk of PAD by over twofold.[247, 255]

In the young, both symptomatic and asymptomatic PAD is more common in men than women but in the elderly there is no gender preference. The annual incidence of claudication has been shown to be 6 per 10,000 for age 30–44-year-old men and 3 per 10,000 for 30–44-year-old women.[251] This same study reported an annual incidence of 61 per 10,000 for 65–74-year-old men and 54 per 10,000 women in this age group.[251]

The presence of coronary artery disease (CAD) triples the risk of developing PAD.[256] Conversely, patients with PAD have a marked increased risk of cardiovascular events, which are related to the severity of the PAD.[256] The overall annual major cardiovascular event rate in patients with PAD is approximately 5–7%.[253] Each 0.1 decrease in the ABI corresponds to a 10% increase of a major cardiovascular event risk.[253]

There is also a strong relationship between PAD severity and mortality. The 5 year all cause mortality rate in patients with PAD is 30%.[253] The 10-year and 15-year all-cause mortality rate in PAD patients are 50% and 70%, respectively.[253] Furthermore, the yearly mortality rate in patients with chronic limb ischemia is 20%, and the short-term amputation risk is 25%.[253] The short-term mortality rate in those patients with acute limb ischemia is 15–20%.[253]

Despite progression of the underlying atherosclerotic process, the clinical course of PAD, however, is surprisingly stable. Only about 25% of claudicants will experience any clinical deterioration.[253] Stable claudication continues in 70–80%, worsening claudication occurs in 10–20%, and critical limb ischemia results in 1–2%.[253]

Nonfatal myocardial infarction or stroke occurs in 20%; death results in 15–30% with three quarters of the resulting deaths being caused by cardiovascular complications.[253] The prognosis is significantly worse in diabetics, hyperlipidemics, and in those who continue to smoke.[253] Only 1–3.3% of patients with claudication require major amputation within 5 years.[253] This clinically stable course has been attributed to the development of collaterals, metabolic muscle adaptation, or to the patient changing his or her lifestyle to favor non-ischemic muscle groups.[253]

On the contrary, the natural history of critical limb ischemia (CLI) and of acute limb ischemia (ALI) is more malignant. It has been documented that nearly 40% of CLI patients will require amputations and at 1 year only 50% of patients are alive.[253, 257] The 30-day amputation rate in ALI patients is 10–30%.[257] It is important to stress that prior to any amputation an anatomic evaluation should always be performed to assess possible revascularization options.

Symptoms of PAD depend on the stenosis severity, the degree of collateral circulation, and the vigor of the exercise. Patients may be asymptomatic (25–50%), experience intermittent claudication, CLI (1–2%) or ALI.[257] A lack of symptoms may be due to physical inactivity. Atypical leg pain is seen in 40–50% of PAD patients while classic claudication is experienced in 10–35%.[257]

The affected muscle group may help localize the stenosis. Buttock and hip pain often suggest aorto-iliac disease. This is called Leriche's syndrome. Thigh pain commonly denotes femoral artery or aorto-iliac disease. Symptoms referable to the upper two-thirds of the calf signify the superficial femoral artery, the lower one-third of the calf indicates the popliteal artery, and foot claudication denotes tibial or peroneal artery disease. Nocturnal leg cramps may mimic PAD but are thought to be neuromuscular in origin.

Typical intermittent claudication is defined as reproducible discomfort of a defined muscle group induced by exercise and relieved by rest. It results from an imbalance between blood supply and tissue demand. It usually results from disease within the inflow and outflow vessels of the lower extremities but may also be due to abdominal aortic disease. Since the natural history of typical intermittent claudication is relatively benign, treatment decisions should be symptom dependent. The Fontaine and Rutherford classification systems[253] (Table 8.1) have been developed to guide a symptomatic treatment approach.

Atypical claudication is defined as pain or discomfort of a particular muscle group that does not require cessation of activity, pain that is not predictable with activity, discomfort that does not resolve within 10 min of rest, or pain at rest and with exertion. Patients with leg pain during exertion and at rest are more likely to be diabetics with true PAD or patients with pseudoclaudication caused by neuropathy or spinal stenosis.[258]

Critical limb ischemia (CLI) describes the condition of PAD patients who suffer from typical chronic ischemic rest pain, including ischemic ulcers and gangrene. While patients with claudication usually have more focal atherosclerotic lesions, patients with CLI are more likely to have diffuse, more distally located atherosclerosis.

ALI denotes any acute decrease in limb perfusion that may threaten limb viability. The signs of ALI include pain, pulselessness, pallor, paresthesias, and paralysis. Mortality

TABLE 8.1. Fontaine and Rutherford classification systems for chronic intermittent claudication.

Fontaine		Rutherford		
Stage	Clinical	Grade	Category	Clinical
I	Asymptomatic	0	0	Asymptomatic
IIa	Mild claudication	I	1	Mild claudication
IIb	Moderate to severe claudication	I	2	Moderate claudication
		I	3	Severe claudication
III	Ischemic rest pain	II	4	Ischemic rest pain
IV	Ulceration or gangrene	III	5	Minor tissue loss
		III	6	Major tissue loss

rates for ALI range from 15% to 20%. Major amputations are required in up to 25%.[253]

Increased compartment pressure may cause calf pressure and tightness. It is seen predominantly in athletes with chronic, repetitive exercise. It may persist even after resting.

Patients with vasospastic claudication will have normal pulses at rest and no bruits. A subcritical underlying stenosis may be associated with vasospasm.

8.2.1.1 Treatment of Peripheral Arterial Atherosclerosis

Stable Intermittent Claudication

To determine the best treatment for claudication, the clinician must assess the interplay among the risks of a specific intervention, the likely degree of expected clinical improvement, and the potential durability of the procedure. The main directives in the treatment of stable intermittent claudication are symptom relief as well as improved exercise tolerance and quality of life. Since treatment decisions for chronic intermittent claudication are symptom based, the Fontaine and Rutherford classification systems[253] mentioned in the preceding pages are quite useful (Table 8.1).

Treatment options include exercise training, medications, percutaneous intervention or surgical revascularization, and amputation. A supervised exercise program often results in improved exercise performance and walking ability.[259] Medications, such as cilostazol (pletal), phosphodiesterase inhibitors, and pentoxifylline (trental) which improves blood flow by decreasing its viscosity, may improve symptoms.[260-263]

Frequently, however, revascularization options are most often utilized in the treatment of intermittent claudication. If the risk–benefit analysis favors revascularization, the most appropriate intervention and technique must be based on a complete evaluation and characterization of the atherosclerotic location, degree, extent, and morphology. Patency following percutaneous transluminal angioplasty (PTA) is highest for lesions in the common iliac artery and progressively decreases for lesions in more distal vessels.

Anatomic factors that affect the duration of patency include severity of disease in run-off arteries, length of the stenosis/occlusion, and the number of lesions treated. Clinical variables impacting the outcome also include diabetes, renal failure, smoking, and the severity of ischemia. Methods to perform the prerequisite anatomic evaluation prior to deciding on a particular treatment include the physical examination, Doppler ultrasound, computed tomographic (CT) angiography, magnetic resonance angiography (MRA), and invasive catheterization. If all factors are equal, clinicians will often choose an endovascular revascularization approach for those patients who have failed a conservative approach.

The TransAtlantic Inter-Society Consensus (TASC) Working Group along with the Society of Interventional Radiologists (SIR) has published a lesion classification system (Tables 8.2 and 8.3).[253] This document classifies PAD according to the level of disease (aorto-iliac and femoral popliteal) and by its severity. It also offers a guide to the most appropriate revascularization approach for each lesion class. As the disease severity worsens, recommendations move from an endovascular to an open surgical approach.

Stable Intermittent Claudication and Aorto-Iliac Atherosclerosis

Severe stenoses in the aorto-iliac region are rare and when present are usually short in length. They are seen more often in obese females and in smokers. In addition, they commonly occur in patients with congenital aortic hypoplasia.[264] Both open and endovascular procedures have 5-year patency rates in the 50% range with acceptable complication rates.[265, 266] Endovascular procedural complications usually relate to embolization and pseudoaneurysm formation. Although aorto-bifemoral bypass appears to have better long-term patency than the currently available endovascular strategies for diffuse aorto-iliac occlusive disease, the risks of surgery are significantly greater than the risks of an endovascular approach in terms of not only mortality but also major morbidity and delay in return to normal activities. Therefore, the

TABLE 8.2. TransAtlantic Inter-Society Consensus (TASC) Working Group classification system for aorto-iliac atherosclerotic lesions.

TASC classification: aorto-iliac lesions

Type A:
– Unilateral or bilateral stenoses of the common iliac artery
– Unilateral or bilateral single short (≤3 cm)

Type B:
– Short (≤3 cm) stenosis of the infrarenal aorta
– Unilateral common iliac artery occlusion
– Single or multiple stenoses totaling 3–10 cm involving the external iliac artery not extending into the common femoral artery
– Unilateral external iliac occlusion not involving the origins of the internal iliac or common femoral artery

Type C:
– Bilateral common iliac occlusions
– Bilateral external iliac stenoses 3–10 cm long not extending into the common femoral artery
– Unilateral external iliac artery occlusion that involves the origins of the internal iliac and or the common femoral artery
– Heavily calcified unilateral external iliac occlusion with or involvement of the origins of the internal iliac and or common femoral artery

Type D:
– Infrarenal aortoiliac occlusion
– Diffuse disease involving the aorta and both iliac arteries requiring treatment
– Diffuse multiple stenoses involving the unilateral common iliac, external iliac and common femoral arteries
– Unilateral occlusions of both the common iliac and external iliac artery
– Bilateral occlusions of the external iliac artery
– Iliac stenoses in patients with AAA requiring treatment and not amenable to endograft placement or other lesions requiring open aortic or iliac surgery

assessment of the patient's general condition and anatomy of the diseased segment(s) are central in deciding which approach is warranted.

The technical and initial clinical success of angioplasty for iliac stenoses exceeds 90% in all reports in the literature.[253] The initial technical success rates approach 100% for focal iliac lesions.[253] For recanalization of long segment iliac

TABLE 8.3. TransAtlantic Inter-Society Consensus (TASC) Working Group classification system for femoral popliteal atherosclerotic lesions.

TASC classification: femoral popliteal lesions

Type A:
- Single stenosis ≤ 10 cm in length
- Single occlusion ≤ 5 cm in length

Type B:
- Multiple lesions (stenoses or occlusions) each ≤ 5 cm
- Single stenosis or occlusion ≤ 15 cm not involving the infrageniculate popliteal artery
- Single or multiple lesions in the absence of continuous tibial vessels to improve inflow for a distal bypass
- Single popliteal stenosis

Type C:
- Multiple stenoses or occlusions totaling > 15 cm with or without heavy calcification
- Recurrent stenoses or occlusions that need treatment after two endovascular interventions

Type D:
- Chronic total occlusions of the common femoral or superficial femoral artery (>20 cm involving the popliteal artery)
- Chronic total occlusion of the popliteal artery and proximal trifurcation vessels

occlusions with or without additional fibrinolysis, the initial procedural success rates approaches 80–85%.[253] The procedural success was higher for stenting, whereas complication rates and 30-day mortality rates did not differ significantly.[253]

For angioplasty alone, investigators have published 5-year patency rates of 72%.[267, 268] The patency for claudicants was nearly 80%.[267, 268] The durability of stenting procedures has been documented with 8-year primary patency rates reported to be in the 74% range.[269] Factors that affect the iliac artery angioplasty and stent patency include the quality of the run-off vessels, the severity of ischemia, and the length of diseased segments. Female gender has also been suggested to decrease patency of external iliac artery stents.[270]

If an endovascular procedure for aorto-iliac disease is considered first, there is only one randomized controlled trial available for guidance in choosing primary stenting versus angioplasty alone with subsequent selective stenting if needed.[271] While 43% of the primary stent group ultimately required stenting, at 2 years, the cumulative patency rate was equal for the two groups (71% for the primary stent cohort versus 70% for the primary angioplasty and selective stenting group). Thus, these authors suggest a primary angioplasty approach followed by stenting only if required. It must be noted that this trial studied mainly short-segment stenoses (<5 cm). There is little guidance available in the literature for the most optimal approach for long (>5 cm) iliac stenoses.

For iliac occlusions, stenting (as opposed to angioplasty alone) is associated with less procedural related complications such as embolization but similar long-term patency as angioplasty alone.[264] The 2-year reintervention rates for angioplasty and for primary stenting were low at 7% and 4% (not significant), respectively.[272] The 5-year freedom from revascularization was also similar at 82% and 80%, respectively.[272]

In a meta-analysis of six articles, Bosch and Hunink compared the results of aorto-iliac angioplasty versus aorto-iliac stenting.[273] Technical success was higher for stenting, whereas complication rates and 30-day mortality rates were similar. In patients with intermittent claudication, the 4-year primary patency rates (adjusted for lesion severity), after excluding technical failures, were 68% for angioplasty and 77% for stenting. The relative risk of long-term failure was reduced by 39% after stent placement compared with angioplasty alone. It is reasonable to expect that the newer techniques and equipment now available would lead to even better results.

In fact, stent design is ever changing. Nitinol (nickel–titanium) is in the unique class of materials known as shape–memory alloys. The superelasticity of nitinol is the most dramatic advantage afforded by this material, but by no means the only one. Nitinol also possesses outstanding corrosion resistance and biocompatibility. Superelasticity refers to the unusual ability of certain metals to undergo large elastic deformation. While many metals exhibit superelastic effects, only nitinol-based alloys appear to be chemically and biologically compatible with the human body. The force applied by a superelastic device is determined by the temperature, not by the strain. Therefore, since the body temperature is for the most part constant, pressure from surrounding tissues has little if any effect on a nitinol stent. In addition, the extraordinary compliance of nitinol clearly makes it the metal that is most similar mechanically to biological materials.

Another unique attribute of superelastic devices is that they can be deployed using the shape–memory effect. The most common superelastic medical devices are these self-expanding nitinol stents. Further advantages of nitinol stents over current balloon-expandable stents include a greater resistance to crushing in exposed vessels (such as the femoral or popliteal areas), lower bending stresses when situated in tortuous paths, more flexible delivery systems, the ability to scaffold cross-sections other than circles, and the elimination of acute recoil.

The outcome of two different self-expanding (nitinol) stents for the treatment of iliac artery lesions has been evaluated.[274] The 1-year primary patencies were 94.7% and 91.1% (not significant), respectively, with similar complication and symptomatic improvement rates regardless of the type of stent.

For symptomatic iliac disease, only one randomized controlled study to date has compared open surgery with angioplasty.[275] Three deaths were reported in the surgery group versus none in the angioplasty cohort. There was no difference in patency or in limb salvage between the two groups within the 4-year follow-up. The authors suggested that the lower morbidity in the percutaneously treated group favors angioplasty as the initial approach if the anatomy is suitable. This suggestion is further supported by the fact that percutaneous techniques and equipment have markedly improved since 1993.

A second, nonrandomized, comparative study evaluated the primary patency rates of stent deployment versus open bypass surgery for iliac lesions and found a significantly better primary patency rate for bypass surgery at 18 months (93% versus 73%), 30 months (93% versus 68%), and 42 months (93% versus 68%).[253] Few data exist regarding primary stenting of aorto-iliac disease. Early angioplasty alone was fraught with embolic complications.

If surgery is contemplated, choice of the appropriate surgical procedure is driven by the particular anatomy and by the expertise of the surgeon. Traditionally, surgical management of a single iliac artery occlusion is with femoral to femoral crossover bypass, especially if the lesion involves the femoral artery. The operative mortality is in the 0–5% range.[276] A 22% complication rate has been reported with a 6% graft infection rate.[277] Unilateral iliofemoral bypass grafting is also a favorable procedure.[277]

Since data comparing surgery with endovascular treatment of aorto-iliac disease are contradictory and since there are no guidelines upon which to rely, the TASC Working Group has published recommendations for treatment of iliac disease. Endovascular treatment should be first line in type A lesions.[253] While the data to support a primary endovascular approach for type B lesions is scarce, the TASC Working Group prefers an endovascular approach first unless an open procedure is required for other associated lesions.[253] Since open revascularization produces superior long-term results, bypass surgery is recommended first in patients with type C lesions unless the risk of surgery is too high.[253] Type D lesions yield poor results with an endovascular approach and thus surgical revascularization is recommended.[253]

Bilateral surgical bypass from the infrarenal abdominal aorta to both femoral arteries is usually recommended for diffuse disease throughout the aorto-iliac segment.[253] The use of polytetrafluoroethylene (PTFE or Teflon) versus Dacron as a conduit in this position is based on the preference of the surgeon. Endarterectomy is not as widely practiced as bypass grafting.[253] Reported 5-year primary patency rates range from 60% to 94% and they are highly operator dependent.[253]

When avoidance of an abdominal approach is necessary, a modified retroperitoneal approach or a unilateral bypass with a femorofemoral crossover may be used.[253] Alternatively in these situations, an axillo-bifemoral or crossover femoral bypass may be considered.[253] Patency rates depend upon the indication for the reconstruction and the justification for the unilateral bypass (normal inflow artery versus high surgical risk).[253] In some cases, patency of a unilateral bypass can be enhanced by endovascular techniques.[253] The thoracic aorta has also been used as an inflow artery.[253]

Stable Intermittent Claudication and Infrainguinal Arterial Atherosclerosis

Femoral and popliteal disease is the most common site for unfavorable anatomy for intervention because this area often has diffuse and heavy calcification. In addition, chronic total occlusions are common and long lesions are often present. Because of this complex disease these locations are prone to high restenosis rates. Furthermore, stents in these areas are exposed to external forces like bending of the knees and hips, which may lead to stent fractures. Given these factors, balloon angioplasty alone is frequently utilized. Plaque excision and cutting balloon angioplasty may be required. When needed, bioabsorbable stents, nitinol stents, and covered stents (more prone to edge restenosis) are used since they more successfully withstand the aforementioned external forces.

When revascularization is considered for infrainguinal disease, a surgical approach has traditionally been the treatment of choice. However, endovascular therapy in these regions for patients with intermittent claudication is well established. Because of the low morbidity and mortality of endovascular therapy in the infrainguinal territory, it is the preferred treatment for stenoses and occlusions up to 10 cm in length.[253] In addition, with the advent of newer techniques and equipment such as blunt dissection devices, cryotherapy, atherectomy devices, cutting balloons, subintimal angioplasty, and stents, percutaneous intervention is used more frequently in the femoral, popliteal, and infrapopliteal regions.

It should be noted that when utilizing an endovascular approach in the infrainguinal region, identification of profunda artery patency is important. Problems with the profunda artery may convert a patient with claudication to a patient with a threatened limb since the profunda artery is often the source for lower extremity collaterals.

Unflawed data regarding stenting and primary angioplasty for infrainguinal lesions are scarce.[264] One-year patency rates of femoral and popliteal stenoses and occlusions after angioplasty are reported at 70% and 50%, respectively.[264] The technical and clinical success rate of infrainguinal angioplasty in all series is greater than 95%.[278] Clinical stage of disease, length of lesion, and outflow disease were most commonly found as independent risk factors for restenosis. Generally, acute angioplasty failure of a superficial femoral artery (SFA) lesion requires stent placement.[250]

Results after stenting (including nitinol stents) are variable.[278,279,280] One randomized trial demonstrated significantly higher primary patency rates with stenting versus angioplasty in femoropopliteal artery TASC A and B lesions at 1 year.[281] In another uncontrolled observational study, 1- and 3-year patency rates after stenting were reported to be 90% and 78%, respectively.[282] These studies should be interpreted with caution since most are industry sponsored. Drug-eluting stents have not been shown to have superior restenosis rates over bare metal stents.[283,284]

Mechanical atherectomy as an adjuvant procedure for endovascular revascularization has had reasonable success. The popliteal artery, in particular, is well suited for atherectomy since it is not favorable for stenting due to its location behind the knee. In planning an atherectomy procedure, it is important to characterize the extent and location of the calcium since atherectomy is more difficult in calcified vessels. If significant calcium exists, the stenosis is likely to be tight in the periphery even if the lumen cannot be visualized.[285] As with angioplasty and stenting, identification of bridging collaterals makes atherectomy significantly more difficult. Ultrasound-guided entry may simplify the procedure.

Kandzari et al.[286] reported an 86% technical success rate for mechanical atherectomy but two-thirds of patients required additional angioplasty and 6% required stenting. At

1 year, the primary and secondary patency rates were 84% and 100% for de novo lesions and 54% and 70% for restenosis lesions, respectively.[287] In patients with critical limb ischemia, Keeling et al[287] reported a 6-month target vessel revascularization rate of 4% and a 6-month amputation rate of 13%. Other studies have shown a 1-year limb salvage rate of 86% with mechanical atherectomy.[285] However, lesions with worse TASC classifications experience poorer outcomes.[288]

Laser atherectomy is a technique that has been shown to be useful in recanalizing long superficial femoral artery occlusions but at a cost of more frequent complications. A 90% success rate for complex superficial femoral artery lesions of 20 cm or more has been demonstrated but the primary and secondary 1-year patency rates are 34% and 76%, respectively. Bosiers et al[289] published that over half of these patients require adjunctive procedures with angioplasty or stenting. One-year primary patency and limb salvage rates for TASC B and C lesions have been shown to be 44% and 55%, respectively.[290]

Another endovascular approach is subintimal angioplasty, which has been performed for some time but has become a more frequently used technique to recanalize total occlusions in critical limb ischemia patients. It creates a subintimal dissection with a wire and in this manner provides blood flow through the occlusion. Technical success has been reported in 87% of patients with primary patency rates of 74% at 1 year.[291]

Clinical success and limb salvage rates at 2 years have been shown to be 72% and 88%, respectively.[292] One study showed similar primary and secondary patency rates between surgical bypass and subintimal angioplasty, but limb salvage at 1 year favored the subintimal angioplasty cohort (97% versus 82%).[293] Procedural complications rates of between 5 and 6% have been reported with subintimal angioplasty.[294]

Cryoangioplasty incorporates cold therapy with balloon angioplasty using liquid nitrous oxide balloon inflation. Extreme cold temperature induces smooth muscle cell apoptosis. Technical success with this technique has been reported to be 85% with 9-month clinical patency and target vessel revascularization rates of 70% and 82%, respectively. At 3 years, clinical patency rates have been reported to be 75%.[295]

On the other hand, cutting balloon angioplasty has achieved 67% and 83% 1-year primary and secondary patency rates, respectively.[296]

Infrapopliteal atherosclerosis is associated with diabetes and is often diffuse in nature. Occlusions are common.[297] Endovascular interventions in the infrapopliteal arteries (peroneal trunk and tibial vessels) are limited to those with severe claudication, rest pain or tissue loss in order to salvage the limb (CLI and ALI patients). The success of these procedures does not justify their use in less severe cases. Procedural success depends on sufficient inflow.[264] In addition, success is less likely in occlusions.[264] Angioplasty of a short anterior or posterior tibial artery stenosis may be performed in conjunction with popliteal or femoral angioplasty.

Predictors of successful endovascular treatment outcomes in the infrapopliteal regions include a shorter length of occlusion and a lesser number of vessels treated.[264] The complication rate (2.4% to 17% depending upon the definition) can usually be treated by endovascular or surgical techniques and a failed angioplasty does not preclude subsequent bypass.[264] It remains controversial whether infrapopliteal angioplasty and stenting should be performed in patients with stable intermittent claudication for improvement of outflow and for an increased patency of proximal angioplasty, stenting, and bypass surgery.

There are very few randomized trials comparing endovascular therapy with bypass surgery in infrainguinal arterial obstructive disease. However, Wolf et al.[298] published a multicenter, prospective, randomized trial comparing angioplasty with open surgical revascularization in patients suffering from iliac, femoral, or popliteal artery obstructions. No significant outcome differences (survival, patency, and limb salvage) were identified in the treatment groups at 4 years.

However, in patients with longer occlusions, the cumulative 1-year primary patency after endovascular therapy was 43% compared with 82% after bypass. This demonstrates that in those patients with long SFA stenoses or occlusions, surgery is better option than angioplasty. The 6-month amputation-free survival rate has been shown to be similar between and endovascular and a surgical approach.

A second, randomized trial (BASIL trial) comparing infrainguinal bypass to endovascular therapy has also been published.[299] The 30-day mortality was 5% and 3% for surgery and angioplasty, respectively. Surgery was associated with more myocardial infarction and wound infection and with longer hospital stays. Those randomized to angioplasty required more future procedures due to recurrence of disease (28% versus 17% at 12 months). No difference was noted in quality of life, amputation-free survival or in all-cause mortality at 2 and 5 years. Subgroup analyses suggest a benefit to surgery if the available vein conduits are suitable for use.

The great saphenous vein is the most optimal conduit for infrainguinal bypass surgery if the vein is large enough (>3 mm diameter).[264] When no vein is available, a vein cuff is recommended at the distal anastomosis of the artificial conduit to promote long-term patency.[300] However, poor long-term patency rates and concerns over graft infection limit the use of prosthetic graft conduits.[301]

Since infrainguinal bypass procedures require adequate inflow to maintain patency, occlusive inflow disease must be identified and corrected prior to proceeding with an outflow surgical procedure. In some situations, a combined approach with dilatation of proximal lesions and surgical bypass of the distal lesions is necessary. If the infrainguinal bypass is constructed following an inflow procedure, patency is improved by making the proximal anastomosis to a native artery rather than the inflow graft (usually, limb of aorto-bifemoral bypass).[302] The quality of the outflow artery is even more important in the maintenance of bypass graft patency than the actual level where the distal anastomosis is performed.[253] The best quality distal vessel should be chosen for the distal anastomosis.

There are currently no large-scale meta-analysis evaluating below-the-knee bypass procedures. Reports have documented 5-year assisted patency rates in vein grafts to approach 60%.[253] In prosthetic below-the-knee bypass grafts, the 5-year assisted patency rates are less than 35%.[253]

Five-year limb salvage rates of 63% and primary patency rates of 41% have been documented in bypass grafts to plantar arteries.[253] In these cases, vein provides better long-term patency than prosthetic graft material.[253] In contrast to the near-equivalent performance of Teflon to vein in above-the-knee bypasses, Teflon performs less well in infrapopliteal grafts (5-year primary and secondary graft patency of 30.5% and 39.7%, respectively).[303] In addition, Teflon graft failures may carry more severe consequences than vein graft failures in this anatomical region.[304] The long saphenous vein (also known as the greater saphenous vein), either in a reversed or in situ configuration offers the best match of size and quality. In its absence, other venous tissue including the contralateral long saphenous vein, short (lesser) saphenous vein, femoral vein or an arm vein should be used.

Differences in surgical outcomes will depend upon the indications for surgery, the quality of the vessels, and the individual patient co-morbidities.[276]

To help guide revascularization decisions, realistic treatment guidelines for infrainguinal atherosclerosis, have been published by the TASC Working Group.[253] Endovascular therapy is the treatment of choice for type A lesions and surgery is the optimal treatment for type D lesions. Endovascular therapy is the treatment of choice for type B lesions and surgery in an adequate risk candidate is recommended for type C lesions. For type B and C lesions, the patient risk and operator expertise are critical in deciding on a primary endovascular or surgical approach. If an endovascular approach is chosen, the specific technique that is utilized is based on the lesion characteristics, the arterial anatomy, the presence of an occlusion or a subtotal stenosis, and on the clinician's judgment and expertise.

Chronic Total Occlusion

Chronic total occlusions (CTO) have historically been difficult to treat percutaneously. Acute procedural success for
endovascular therapy in CTO has improved greatly with
newer equipment, specialized devices, and techniques. Newer
devices (hydrophilic guide wires) and technical improvements (subintimal recanalization) provide high technical success rates in total occlusions of more than 85%.[302] However,
a significant challenge in the treatment of CTOs is the maintenance of long-term patency.

Angioplasty alone is usually suboptimal in CTO because
of large plaque burdens and calcifications. Restenosis due to
neointimal hyperplasia is more common than in subtotal
occlusions or less severe stenoses. Self-expanding nitinol
stents have become more important to prevent elastic recoil
and to stabilize device-induced dissections. Restenosis rates
with nitinol stents, however, is as high as 67%.[253] Patency
rates for CTOs vary depending on the occlusion location, the
length of the occlusion and the presence of calcification.
Stent fracture is still a potential problem.

The overall technical success rate for crossing a CTO with
a guidewire in aorto-iliac and femoropopliteal disease is
reported to be between 71% and 87%.[257,273] Re-entry devices
are best suited for vessels that are not heavily calcified and in
cases where the distal vessel is well visualized.[306] These
devices are useful in cases that have failed an attempt to cross
with the guidewire alone. Perforation is a possible complication. The technical success of subintimal angioplasty also
depends on less calcification and on the presence of a normal
vessel above and below the occlusion to allow proper access
and to increase procedural success.[307]

Blunt microdissection catheters and radiofrequency abla-
tion have also been studied. Success with both procedures
after guidewire failure has been reported.[308] Success rates for
both procedures have been reported in the 75% range.[308]

Complete aortic occlusions are most optimally treated by
an aorto-bifemoral bypass. In a poor surgical candidate, consideration may be given to stenting of the aorta and one iliac

vessel with a femoral to femoral crossover bypass procedure.[309] This approach poses less patient risk but has lower long-term patency rates than an axillary to femoral bypass, which is associated with a 5% in-hospital mortality rate, a 35% five-year patient survival rate and a 75% five-year limb salvage rate.[310] No difference in patency rates is reported between axillary single femoral bypass and axillary bifemoral bypass.[311] For axillary bifemoral bypasses, a flow splitter graft yields better patency rates than a unifemoral bypass with contralateral limb take-off for the continuation to the other limb (86% versus 38%).[311]

Femoropopliteal occlusions are more common than aorto-iliac occlusions and occur more frequently in young, female smokers.[312] They have been reported to be present in 80% of symptomatic patients undergoing angiography.[312] It has been suggested that the frequency of femoropopliteal occlusions is due to the linearity of flow and the relatively few branches in these segments.[313] In addition, torsion and stretching resulting from limb movement has been proposed to be causative.[313]

Chronic and Acute Limb Ischemia

While the treatment for stable intermittent claudication focuses on symptom relief, the primary goals in the treatment of CLI and ALI are pain relief, ulcer healing, limb loss prevention, improved quality of life, and prolonged survival. Contrary to the natural history of stable intermittent claudication, the malignant clinical progression of CLI and ALI mandate treatment attempts to salvage the limb if possible.

In CLI, multi-level disease is frequently encountered. Adequate inflow must be established prior to improvement in the outflow. The successful treatment of a foot ulcer depends on successfully increasing the perfusion to the foot. The determination of whether or not a revascularization procedure is possible will set the tone for the ensuing treatment. There is increasing evidence to support a recommendation for angioplasty in patients with CLI and infrapopliteal artery occlusion where in-line flow to the foot can be re-established and where there is medical co-morbidity. In the case of infrapopliteal angioplasty, technical success may approach 90% with resultant clinical success of approximately 70% in some series of patients with CLI.[253]

In ALI, immediate revascularization is indicated. In those with resulting profound sensory and motor deficits of very short duration, prompt revascularization (within a few hours of symptom onset) may produce complete recovery. Without prompt revascularization, major permanent neuromuscular damage may result. Whether open surgical or endovascular revascularization is attempted depends on the anatomic location of the occlusion, the etiology of ALI, and on the existence of contraindications to open surgical repair.

The immediate goal of treatment for ALI is to prevent thrombus propagation and worsening ischemia. Therefore, immediate anticoagulation with heparin is indicated. Stenoses and occlusions are rarely the sole cause of ALI or even severe chronic symptoms but these commonly lead to superimposed thrombosis and, therefore, should be treated to avoid recurrent thrombosis. Based on the results of randomized trials, there is no clear superiority for systemic thrombolysis versus surgery on 30-day limb salvage or mortality.[253] However, catheter-directed thrombolytic therapy in the treatment of ALI may be beneficial.[253] Published data from randomized, prospective, controlled trials in ALI patients do suggest that catheter-directed thrombolysis may be advantageous over initial surgical revascularization.[253] Patients undergoing catheter-directed thrombolysis experience reduced mortality rates and subsequently require less complex surgical procedures.[253]

In addition, it appears that reperfusion with catheter-directed thrombolysis is achieved at a lower pressure and may result in less reperfusion injury compared to open surgery.[253] However, a catheter-directed thrombolysis approach may result in higher failure rates, more persistent and recurrent ischemia, more major complications, and ultimately, more amputations.[253] Thus, catheter-directed thrombolysis should only be considered initially if the limb is not immediately or irreversibly threatened since it may then offer a lower risk revascularization option.

In cases of acute suprainguinal occlusion (no femoral pulse) open surgery may be preferred since catheter embolectomy is not very effective in removing frequently present, large common iliac artery or distal aortic emboli.[253] Suprainguinal graft occlusion may be best treated with surgery as well.[253] Infrainguinal causes of ALI (embolism or thrombosis), are most often optimally treated with an endovascular approach.[253] Frequently, catheter-based thrombolysis precedes more permanent revascularization since the underlying occlusive disease may be revealed and an appropriate, more permanent adjunctive procedure may be selected.

When treating late, acute graft thrombosis, the main goals are to remove the clot and correct the underlying lesion that caused the thrombosis. The TASC Working Group[253] recommends that in most patients, at least one attempt to salvage a graft should be attempted. Patients should be considered on a case-by-case basis. In cases where atherosclerotic progression results in worsened blood flow in the inflow or outflow vessels, corrective angioplasty, stenting or bypass grafting is also performed.

Treatment for intrinsic graft lesions depends on the type of conduit. Venous bypass grafts often develop stenoses at the site of a valve and may be best suited for thrombolysis followed by angioplasty, stenting or surgical revision.[253] Surgical revision often leads to the most optimal long-term results.[253] Prosthetic grafts frequently develop intimal hyperplasia at the distal anastomosis.[253] These lesions respond less well to angioplasty alone and often require adjunctive stenting.[253]

Figures 8.4–8.30 are examples of peripheral arterial atherosclerotic disease, stents, bypass grafting, and complications from corrective procedure attempts.

Screening for Peripheral Arterial Disease

All patients with exertional leg symptoms should undergo ankle-brachial indices (ABI) and if abnormal, a duplex Doppler ultrasound. In addition, ABI evaluations should take place in patients age 50–69 years who have cardiovascular risk

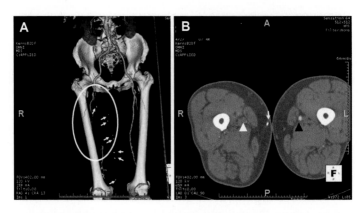

FIGURE 8.4. Panel A is a demonstration of a volume-rendered, segmented image depiction of a long right femoral artery occlusion (*white circle*). The *small white arrows* highlight the clips that mark the course of an occluded right femoral to popliteal venous bypass graft. Panel B is a multiplanar reformat demonstrating the occluded superficial femoral artery (*white arrow head*). The patent left superficial femoral artery is marked by the *black arrow head*. The *white arrow* highlights a bypass clip to the occluded femoral to popliteal venous graft.

factors. Patients greater than 70 years of age, regardless of risk factor status, should also have an ABI evaluation. Furthermore, ABIs should be performed on all diabetics age 40 years or greater and also on those patients with known CAD, cerebrovascular disease (CVD), or renal artery disease. In addition, all patients with a Framingham risk score of greater than 10% should have an ABI examination.[257]

Patients who have undergone peripheral arterial endovascular procedures require careful long-term follow-up to detect recurrences and new progression of disease. The possibility of recurrence remains for a lifetime. The recommended frequency of follow-up depends on disease burden, location, and type of procedure but must be individualized. Aortic and common iliac procedures have less recurrence than infrainguinal procedures and may require less surveillance. Infrainguinal surgery or percutaneous treatment have

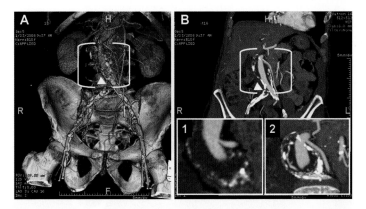

FIGURE 8.5. An aneurysmal distal abdominal aorta (*white brackets* in panels A and B) with an occluded ostial right common iliac artery (*white arrow heads* in panels A and B). There are collaterals filling the right external iliac artery. Panel A is a volume rendered reconstruction. The abdominal aortic aneurysm is marked by the white brackets. The right common iliac artery occlusion is noted by the *white arrow head*. The aorta and iliac vessels are highly calcified. Panel B and its insets (1 and 2) demonstrate the aortic aneurysm (*white brackets*) with its thrombus and displaced calcium. Insets 1 and 2 are magnifications of the aneurysm. The thrombosed ostial right common iliac artery is marked with a *white arrow head*. Collateral vessels are noted as well which fill the distal right leg circulation.

high restenosis and graft failure rates and require more vigilant surveillance.

In addition to the standard interval history and physical examination, surveillance with Doppler ultrasound is recommended after aorto-iliac and infrainguinal endovascular procedures. A reasonable surveillance approach for aorto-iliac disease includes a Doppler evaluation at baseline after the procedure, at 6 months, at 12 months and then annually. For infrainguinal endovascular procedures, a common surveillance approach includes a Doppler at baseline after the procedure, at 3 months, at 6 months, at 9 months, at 12 months, and then annually.[257]

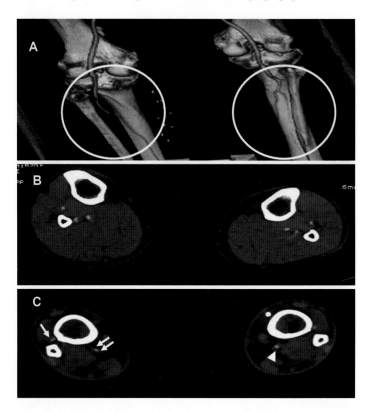

FIGURE 8.6. Illustration of an example of atherosclerosis of the distal run off vessels. Panel A is volume-rendered image suggesting run off disease by the poorly visualized run off vessels (*white circles*). Panel B is a multiplanar reformat (MPR) in the axial plane below the trifurcation of the anterior tibial, posterior tibial and peroneal arteries. All three vessels in each leg are visualized. Panel C is a MPR in an axial plane more caudal than the one in panel B. Here, the right leg demonstrates only the anterior tibial (*single arrow*) and posterior tibial (*double arrow*) arteries. The peroneal artery is absent. The left leg clearly shows only the posterior tibial artery (*arrow head*). The peroneal artery is absent and the anterior tibial artery is barely visualized.

After infrainguinal bypass grafting one suggested surveillance approach consists of a clinical surveillance program immediately after surgery, and at regular 6-month intervals. Clinical

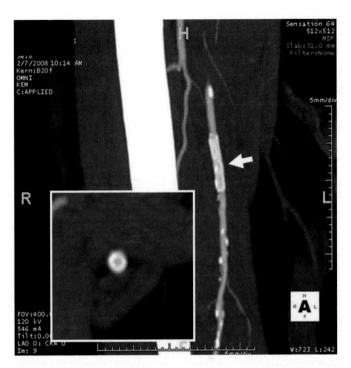

FIGURE 8.7. Demonstration of a patent right superficial femoral artery stent in a maximum intensity projection format (white arrow). The magnified inset is a multiplanar reformat (MPR) in one axial plane through the stent demonstrating full contrast throughout the lumen in this plane. The native femoral vessel has significant calcified and noncalcified plaque, which results in no significant stenoses. Axial MPR is used as a confirmatory tool.

surveillance should include follow-up interval histories to elicit new symptoms, repeated vascular examinations of the legs with palpation of proximal, graft and outflow vessel pulses, periodic measurements of resting and, if possible, post-exercise ABI.

While duplex Doppler ultrasound evaluations after infrainguinal bypass grafting have never been shown to be cost-effective or of clinical benefit,[334,335] many clinicians routinely perform interval (baseline, 3 months, 6 months, 9 months, 12 months and annually) Doppler evaluations to preemptively identify lesions that predispose to graft thrombosis and to allow their repair prior to graft occlusion.[254] Alternatively, Doppler evaluation may be reserved for the onset of new symptoms of claudication or changes in the physical examination.

8.2.2 Popliteal Entrapment Syndrome

Popliteal entrapment syndrome is an important but infrequent cause of claudication and leg pain and may potentially result in disabling symptoms. It is caused by an anomalous

→

FIGURE 8.8. (a) Volume-rendered depiction of multiple stents in the right common and external iliac vessels (*multiple white arrow heads*). A stent is also noted in the left external iliac artery (*single white arrow head*). The distal aorta and the iliac arteries after the bifurcation are highly calcified. The vessels distal to the stents demonstrate good contrast filling. *R* Right, *L* Left, *F* Foot, *H* Head. (b) Representation of curved multiplanar reformats (cMPR) from the patient in (a). Panels A and B are cMPR illustrations through the distal aorta and right iliac stents (Panel A) and distal aorta and left iliac stent (Panel B). The magnified insets (1–5) to the right of panels A and B are magnified axial multiplanar reformats (MPR) in the axial planes marked by the *white arrows*. The stents in panel A are patent but the magnified insets demonstrate more detail. In panel A, inset 1 demonstrates a highly calcified but unobstructed distal aorta. Panel A, inset 2 shows a severe stenosis of the ostial, right common iliac artery (mixed lesion). Panel A, insets 3 and 4 are selected axial planes through the stents highlighting adequate contrast. However, panel A, inset 5 shows a severe stenosis in the distal portion of the stent extending into the native vessel. Panel B shows the left iliac system. Panel A, inset 1 demonstrates unobstructed calcified atherosclerosis in the proximal common iliac artery. Panel B, inset 2 shows a probable tight mixed stenosis. Panel B, inset 3 depicts an entirely calcified lesion obscuring the arterial lumen (probably, a significant lesion). Panel B, inset 4 demonstrates stent patency and panel B, inset 5 depicts a severe obstruction of the vessel distal to the stent. The artery even more distally is subtotally occluded. MPR is used to provide more detail and increase reading accuracy.

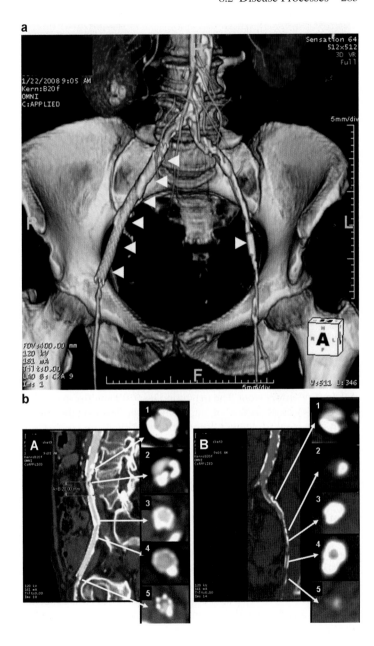

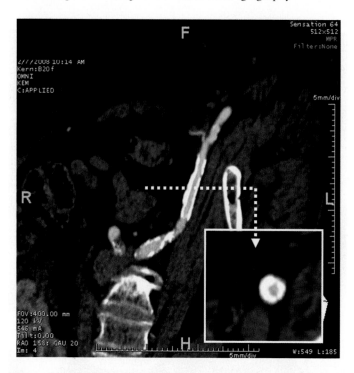

FIGURE 8.9. Maximum intensity projection (MIP) of a left superficial femoral artery stent. The magnified inset is a multiplanar reformat (MPR) cross-section of the stent at the level of the dotted arrow. The stent is patent. Cross-sectional MPR is used to confirm what is seen in MIP reformats.

relationship between the popliteal artery and the surrounding anatomic structures. First described in 1879[313], it usually occurs in younger patients without risk factors for atherosclerosis.[313] It is most often seen in athletes participating in soccer, basketball, and rugby since these sports often result in hypertrophy of the gastrocnemius muscle.[313]

There are three requisite conditions that must coexist for popliteal artery entrapment syndrome to occur.[313] First, there must be an abnormal anatomical relationship between the popliteal artery and the surrounding muscles and tendons.

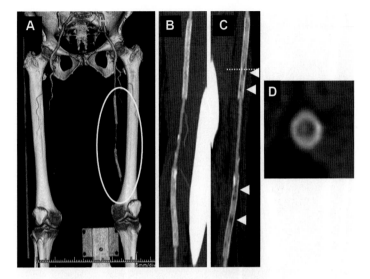

FIGURE 8.10. Demonstration of the importance of utilizing multiple reformatting (MPR) techniques to provide a diagnosis. Panel A is a volume rendered, segmented image identifying the two superficial femoral artery stents *circled in white*. Panel B is a maximum intensity projection (MIP) of the same stented regions which falsely depicts no obvious problems. However, panel C is a curved multiplanar reformat of the same stents demonstrating multiple regions of severe in-stent stenosis. Panel D is a cross-sectional MPR at the level of the dotted line in panel C further showing the severity of the in-stent stenosis in this location. MPR is mandatory for better evaluating within stents and other problem areas. Diagnoses are never made solely on volume rendered and MIP images alone.

Second, hypertrophy of the muscles and tendons must occur. Lastly, recurrent compression of the arterial must occur with exercise.

Multiple anatomic variants of popliteal entrapment syndrome have been observed. There may be an atypical course of the popliteal artery.[314] A normally coursing popliteal artery may be compressed by hypertrophy of an anomalous gastrocnemius muscles.[315] In this case, the two heads of the gastrocnemius muscle often lie in an anterior and posterior location

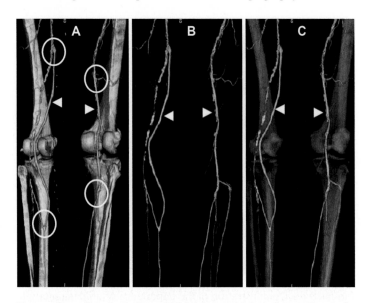

FIGURE 8.11. Panels A, B, and C depict multiple reformatting techniques illustrating the peripheral vasculature. Here, bilateral femoral popliteal bypass grafts (*white arrow heads*) are noted in a segmented volume rendered reconstruction (Panel A), a segmented volume rendered image with bone subtraction (Panel B) and with a semitransparent depiction of the bones (Panel C). The proximal and distal anastomoses are circled in white (Panel A) (Reproduced with kind permission from the Radiological Society of North America. Copyright 2008. Lopera J, Trimmer C, Josephs S, et al. Multidector CT angiography of infrainguinal arterial bypass. *Radiographics*. 2008;28:529–549).

instead of lying side-by-side as they usually do. Finally, a combination of an anomalous popliteal artery, a mislocated artery or a muscular abnormality may occur.[314] Uncommonly, the popliteal vein, rather than the popliteal artery, is involved.[314] Hai et al. have proposed a classification system for this entity (Table 8.4).[315]

Because of the repetitive popliteal artery compressions, resulting arterial pathology such as poststenotic dilation, true aneurysm formation, and thrombosis at the site of entrapment

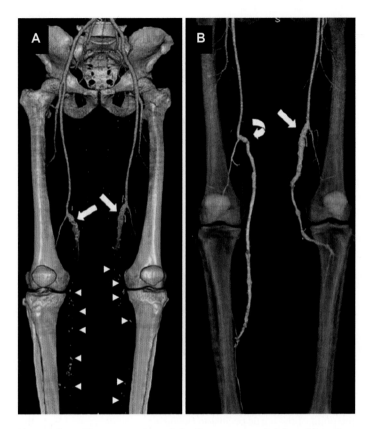

FIGURE 8.12. Demonstration of the importance of delayed imaging. This patient has undergone a right femoral tibial bypass graft and a left femoral popliteal bypass. The patient was evaluated for claudication. Panel A depicts poor filling of the bypass grafts (*white arrows*). The *white arrow heads* point out the clips marking the course of the bypass grafts. Panel B is a delayed image showing adequate visualization and filling of both bypass grafts (*curved and strait arrows*) (Reproduced with kind permission from the Radiological Society of North America. Copyright 2008. Lopera J, Trimmer C, Josephs S, et al. Multidector CT angiography of infrainguinal arterial bypass. *Radiographics*. 2008;28:529–549).

may ensue.[315] Extensive collateral development is frequently present.[311]

It is noteworthy that entrapment syndromes may occur at other arterial levels. For example, the inguinal ligament may constrict the iliac artery.

a

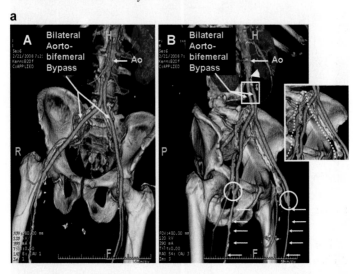

FIGURE 8.13. (a) Illustration of a segmented, volume rendered image of an aorto-bifemoral bypass with bilateral femoral popliteal extensions. Panels A and B depict the bypass grafts emanating from the point of the aortic occlusion (*white arrow head* in panel B) to the bilateral superficial femoral arteries. The distal anastomoses from the aorto-bifemoral connection and from the proximal anastomoses of the femoral popliteal connections are within the white circles in panel B. The occluded segment of the aorta is within the white square in panel B. The magnified inset of panel B highlights the native calcified distal aorta after the long occlusion and the calcified, severely diseased bilateral common iliac arteries (*dotted white lines*). The white arrows in panel B depict the femoral to popliteal bypass graft extensions. (b) From the patient in Fig. 8.13a. Here panel A shows the distal anastomoses of the graft with the popliteal artery (*circled in white* and magnified in the insets below panel A). Panel B demonstrates the bilateral proximal anastomoses of the femoral popliteal extensions (white circles). The magnified insets above panel B better depict these latter anastomoses. The *white arrows* in panels A and B depict the clips from the harvested veins.

b

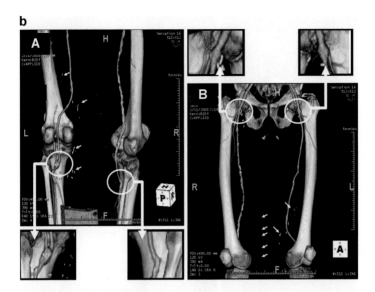

FIGURE 8.13. (continued).

Popliteal artery entrapment syndrome is uncommon and difficult to diagnose. Awareness of this syndrome is crucial to making an accurate diagnosis since clinical suspicion is the first step and a careful history and physical examination are necessary. Symptoms and signs may vary and include leg swelling, aching pain, pain at rest, and tiredness or cramping of the calf. Symptoms at rest may be absent prior to the development of complications. Early on, patients may note transitory cramps and coolness of the leg. Numbness, pallor, coolness, and cramping may occur in some postures and resolve with changing position. The symptoms may be sudden and severe during physical exercise. Acute ischemia may occur later if thrombosis occurs.[315] Often, a provocative maneuver during physical examination is required such as extension of the foot and contraction of the calf. This maneuver may result in a diminished or absent popliteal pulse.

Traditionally, bilateral invasive angiography has been the gold standard for diagnosing popliteal entrapment syndrome. Possible angiographic signs include internal deviation of the

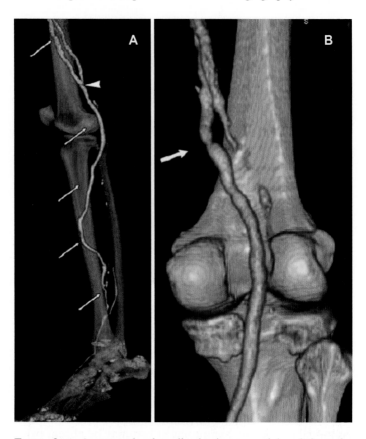

FIGURE 8.14. An example of a spliced vein sequential graft from the mid superficial femoral artery to the anterior tibial artery. Three segments of the cephalic and basilica veins were sewn together to create a longer graft (*thin white arrows* in panel A). The arrow head in panel A depicts a potential moderate stenosis within the vein graft better seen in panel B (*white arrow*) (Reproduced with kind permission from the Radiological Society of North America. Copyright 2008. Lopera J, Trimmer C, Josephs S, et al. Multidector CT angiography of infrainguinal arterial bypass. *Radiographics*. 2008;28:529–549).

popliteal artery as well as a pinched, angulated or narrowed appearance of the popliteal artery. Poststenotic dilatation may also be seen. Partial lesions are classic and demonstrate no evidence for atherosclerotic stenoses elsewhere in the

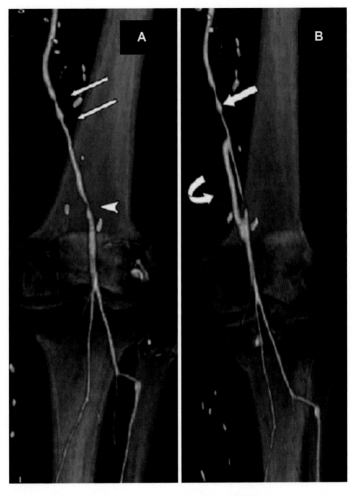

FIGURE 8.15. Depiction of a segmented, volume-rendered, semi-transparent image of a femoral to popliteal bypass. Panel A shows multiple problem areas both proximally (*thin arrows*) and distally (*arrow head*). The distal stenosis was corrected with another short bypass segment (*curved arrow* in panel B). The more proximal advanced graft disease (*thick white arrow* in panel B) required repeat bypass at a later date (Reproduced with kind permission from the Radiological Society of North America. Copyright 2008. Lopera J, Trimmer C, Josephs S, et al. Multidetector CT angiography of infrainguinal arterial bypass. *Radiographics.* 2008;28:529–549).

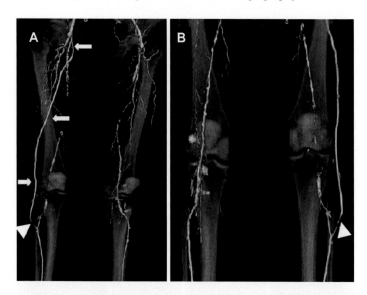

FIGURE 8.16. Demonstration of a right femoral to popliteal bypass graft using a segmented, volume-rendered, semitransparent reconstruction. The bypass graft is noted by the *white arrows* in panel A. A tight distal stenosis is suggested (*white arrow head* in panel A). Note the bilateral, severely diseased native vessels with extensive collateralization. Panel B is a posterior view with the worrisome distal graft segment depicted by the *white arrow head* (Reproduced with kind permission from the Radiological Society of North America. Copyright 2008. Lopera J, Trimmer C, Josephs S, et al. Multidector CT angiography of infrainguinal arterial bypass. *Radiographics.* 2008;28:529–549).

FIGURE 8.17. Demonstration of a femoral to to popliteal bypass graft with stenoses both proximally and distally. Panel A is a volume-rendered, segmented, semitransparent computed tomographic (CT) angiography image and panel B is a conventional angiogram. The straight white arrow in panel A points to a severe stenosis just proximal to the proximal anastomosis. This stenosis is confirmed by conventional angiography (*black straight arrow*). The *curved arrows* depict the CT and conventional angiographic depictions of the critical stenosis just distal to the distal anastomosis. Note the extensive collaterals seen in panel B, which are not well appreciated in panel A (Reproduced with kind permission from the Radiological Society of North America. Copyright 2008. Lopera J, Trimmer C, Josephs S, et al. Multidector CT angiography of infrainguinal arterial bypass. Radiographics. 2008;28:529–549).

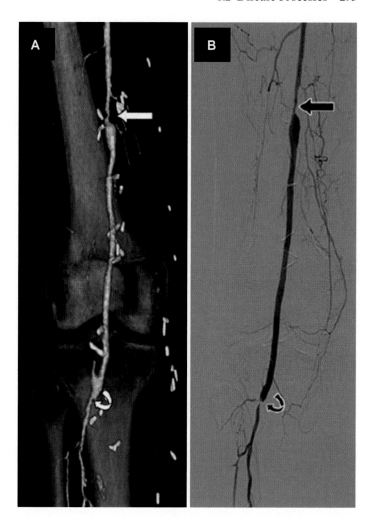

vascular tree. The diagnosis can be confirmed by dynamic arteriography with run-off during calf contraction. If these dynamic maneuvers result in deviation or occlusion of the proximal popliteal artery, the diagnosis is confirmed.[315]

Computed tomographic (CT) angiography may also be used to make this diagnosis. A combined imaging approach including dynamic CT angiography with Doppler examination may be necessary. CT angiography for the diagnosis of popliteal artery entrapment syndrome is relatively new since improvements in CT-scanner technology have only recently been introduced. Advantages of CT angiography include the ability to view and manipulate a three-dimensional data set, allowing exquisite visualization of the soft tissue anatomy in relation to the arterial structures. As with invasive angiography, CT acquisition with contrast administration during submaximal calf muscle contraction may be useful.[315]

The treatment of choice for popliteal artery entrapment syndrome is the surgical creation of normal anatomy within the popliteal fossa.

Figures 8.31 and 8.32 are examples of popliteal entrapment.

8.2.3 Peripheral Arterial Aneurysms

Peripheral arterial aneurysms are often coexistent with abdominal aortic aneurysms (AAA). Up to 85% of patients with femoral artery aneurysms and 62% of those with popliteal aneurysm have a coexistent AAA.[316, 317] Conversely, femoral or popliteal artery aneurysms are present in 3–6% of

---

FIGURE 8.18. (a) An example of a left femoral to popliteal bypass. The volume-rendered, segmented image with bone subtraction in panel A shows the proximal and distal anastomoses of the graft (*white arrow heads*). The right femoral artery is severely diseased. Panel B is a maximum intensity projection pointing out two of the many problem areas in the right femoral system (*white arrows*). Panel C is a magnification of panel A. The white arrow head points to the proximal graft anastomosis. (b) Panels A and B are maximum intensity projections of the proximal (Panel A) and distal (Panel B) graft anastomoses from the patient in Fig. 8.18a. These anastomoses are widely patent.

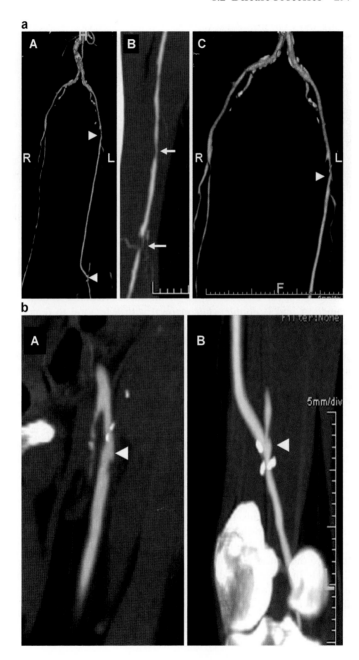

a
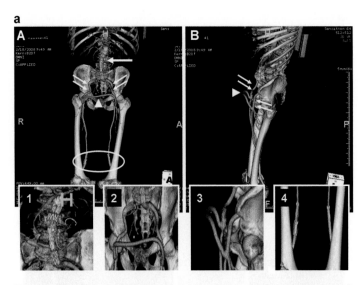

Figure 8.19. (a) Demonstration of an aorto-bifemoral endograft (Panels A and B *double white arrows*) with a femoral to femoral crossover connection (Panels A and B *white arrow head*) and stents in the bilateral distal superficial femoral arteries (*white circle* in panel A). There is also an abdominal aortic stent noted (panel A *white arrow*). Panel A is a segmented, volume-rendered depiction in the anterior view and panel B shows an oblique view. Inset 1 is a magnification of the aortic stent graft. Inset 2 is a magnification of the aorto-bifemoral connection and the femoral to femoral cross-over in the anterior plane. The same is visualized in inset 3 in an oblique plane. Inset 4 is a magnification of the superficial femoral artery stents. (b) Panels A and B are maximum intensity projections nicely depicting the distal anastomoses of the femoral to femoral crossover graft to the native femoral arteries from the patient in Fig. 8.19a. Panel B is a magnification of panel A. (c) highlights the femoral artery stents from the patient in (a). Panel A highlights these stents within the white square in this volume rendered, segmented depiction. Panel B demonstrates the poor distal run-off distal to these stents (within the ovals). The magnified insets further illustrate the stent in a 3-dimensional image (*left*) and in a multiplanar reformatted axial image (*right*), which confirms stent patency at this level.

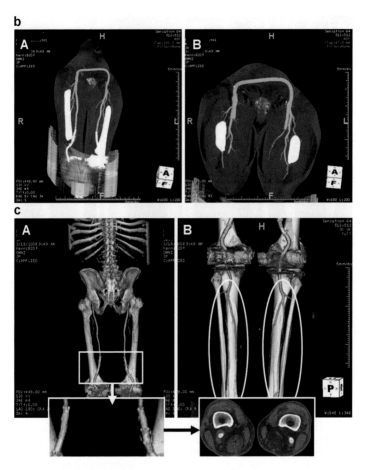

FIGURE 8.19. (contiued).

patients with AAA. Given this association, some have proposed a genetic component. Accordingly, all patients presenting with peripheral arterial aneurysms should be carefully
evaluated for other aneurysms especially in the aorto-iliac
segments and in the other limb. In contrast to aortic aneurysms, the natural history of lower extremity artery aneurysms is that of thromboembolism or thrombosis and not
rupture.

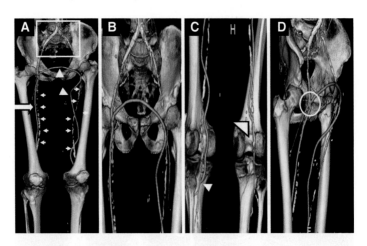

FIGURE 8.20. Illustration of volume-rendered, segmented depictions of a left femoral popliteal venous graft (*white block arrow with black outline* in panel A) with a right femoral to left popliteal crossover venous graft (*large white arrow heads* in panel A). The small arrows in panel A mark the course of the severely calcified and diseased native vessels. The native, severely calcified aorto-iliac region is noted within the white square in panel A. Panel B is a magnification of panel A. Panel C nicely depicts the distal popliteal anastomoses (*white arrow head and white arrow head outlined in black*). Panel D demonstrates the proximal anastomosis of the crossover graft (*white circle*).

FIGURE 8.21. Depiction of volume rendered, segmented images of a right to left femoral to femoral crossover graft (*thin white vertical arrows* in panel A) with an occluded left iliac artery (*white arrow heads* in panel A) and a right iliac stent (*thick white arrow* in panel A). Panel B further depicts the stent (*thick white arrow*) and the left iliac occlusion (*white arrow heads*). The insets in panel B are maximum intensity projections of the anastomoses highlighted by the white squares in the volume rendered image. The proximal anastomosis (*upper inset*) has a severe stenosis. The distal anastomosis (*lower inset*) is widely patent.

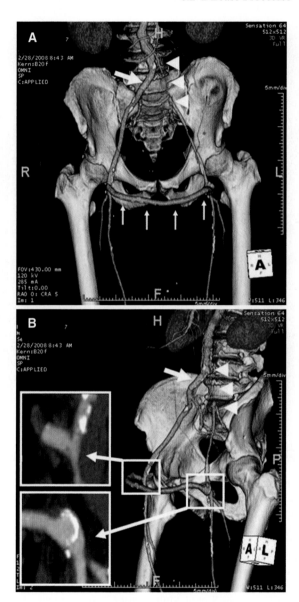

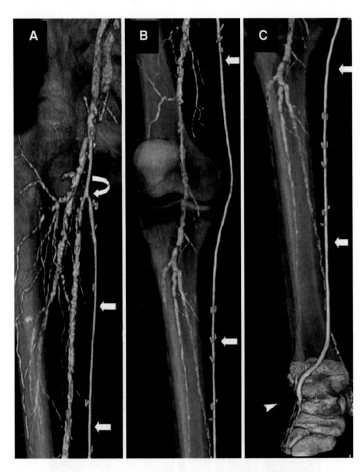

FIGURE 8.22. A normally appearing femoral to popliteal bypass with severely diseased and collateralized native vessels. The images are segmented, volume-rendered, semitransparent reconstructions. Panel A shows the proximal anastomosis nicely (*curved arrow*). The straight white arrows in all panels point to the body of the graft. The arrow head in panel C highlights the distal anastomosis to the popliteal artery (Reproduced with kind permission from the Radiological Society of North America. Copyright 2008. Lopera J, Trimmer C, Josephs S, et al. Multidector CT angiography of infrainguinal arterial bypass. Radiographics. 2008;28:529–549).

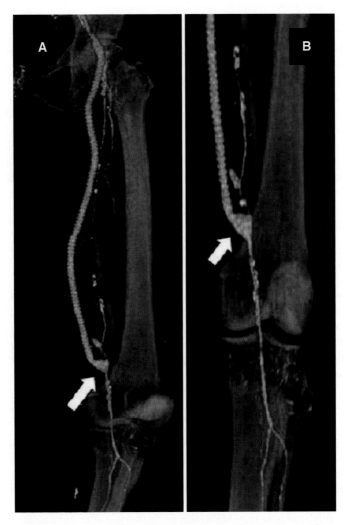

FIGURE 8.23. A volume-rendered, segmented, semitransparent reconstruction of a normal gortex femoral popliteal graft with a cuff of
vein at the anastomosis to the popliteal artery (*white arrows in panels
A and B*)). Panel B is a magnification of panel A. The Gortex graft
has a corrugated appearance (Reproduced with kind permission
from the Radiological Society of North America. Copyright 2008.
Lopera J, Trimmer C, Josephs S, et al. Multidector CT angiography of
infrainguinal arterial bypass. *Radiographics.* 2008;28:529–549).

8.2.3.1 Iliac Artery Aneurysms

Isolated iliac artery aneurysms are rare. They are most commonly associated with AAA. The incidence of iliac artery aneurysms is 0.03–0.1%. Most are asymptomatic but symptoms may occur due to compression, embolization, and rupture. Repair is recommended when symptoms ensue and when the size is 3.5 cm or greater or when there is a rapid increase in diameter (>0.5 cm per year). These aneurysms may be treated surgically or by endovascular exclusion via stenting, which has shown 100% patency rate at 1 year, 97.4% at 2 years, 94.9% at 3 years, and 87.6% at 4 years.[318]

Figure 8.33 demonstrates an extensive right iliac artery aneurysm.

8.2.3.2 Femoral Artery Aneurysms

Femoral artery aneurysms are rare. When present they are usually confined to the common femoral artery. In 50% of the cases the aneurysm may extend to the femoral artery bifurcation. Nearly 85% of all femoral artery aneurysms occur in men. Sixty-nine percent are associated with aortic or iliac aneurysms.[319] Fifty-four percent are contiguous with common

---

FIGURE 8.24. Depiction of a right femoral popliteal bypass (*white arrows* in panel D) and an occluded left superficial femoral artery stent (*arrow head* in panel D). The distal right run-off vessels fill nicely via the bypass graft. There is adequate run-off to the distal vessels in the left leg via collaterals from the profunda artery (*white circle* in panel D). Panel A shows the bypass graft in the axial plane multiplanar reformat (MPR) reconstruction just after its bifurcation (*white arrow*). Panels B and C are also axial MPR reconstructions demonstrating the more superficially coursing graft (*white arrows*). The arrow head in panel B illustrates the occluded left superficial femoral artery stent (Reproduced with kind permission from the Radiological Society of North America. Copyright 2008. Lopera J, Trimmer C, Josephs S, et al. Multidector CT angiography of infrainguinal arterial bypass. *Radiographics*. 2008;28:529–549.

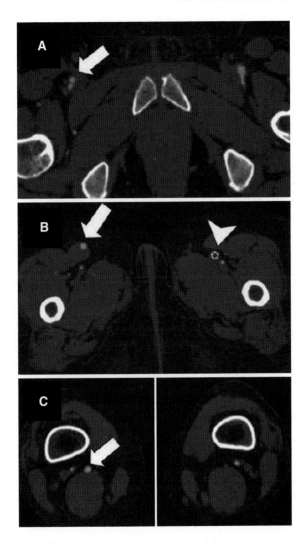

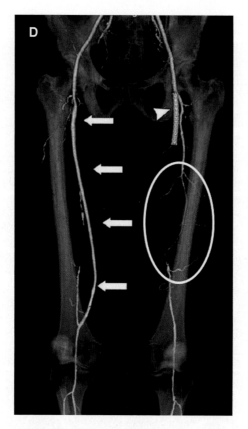

FIGURE 8.24. (continued).

femoral or popliteal artery aneurysms. Isolated aneurysms of
the deep femoral artery are rare and are usually found in
conjunction with an adjacent common femoral artery
aneurysm.[320]

Cutler and Darling proposed a femoral artery aneurysm
classification system.[321] Type I denotes that the aneurysm is
confined to common femoral artery. Type II is when there is
involvement of the orifice of the profunda femoris. This
scheme is useful to aid in operative repair techniques since
type II femoral artery aneurysms may be more difficult to
correct and may require more extensive surgical reconstruction. Femoral artery aneurysms confined to the superficial

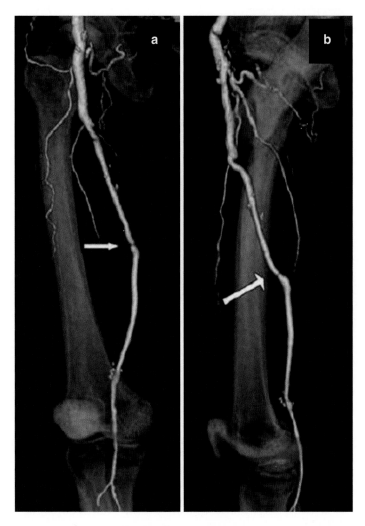

FIGURE 8.25. A volume-rendered, segmented, semitransparent reconstruction nicely depicting a stenosis in the middle portion of a femoral popliteal vein graft. Panel A is an anterior view and panel B is a lateral view. The stenosis was caused by a retained valve cusp. This type of problem usually requires repeat bypass surgery (Reproduced with kind permission from the Radiological Society of North America. Copyright 2008. Lopera J, Trimmer C, Josephs S, et al. Multidector CT angiography of infrainguinal arterial bypass. *Radiographics*. 2008;28:529–549.

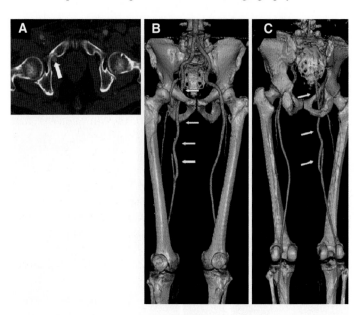

FIGURE 8.26. Depiction of a right iliac to femoral bypass graft using a gortex endoprosthesis. This graft is seen coursing through the obturator foramen which is an unusual anatomic course for this graft, which usually is placed anterior to the pubis. In this case, the patient had a pseudoaneurysm and a non-healing superficial ulcer secondary to radiation treatment for melanoma. Panel A shows a multiplanar reformat with the graft coursing through the obturator foramen. Panels B (anterior) and C (posterior) demonstrate a volume-rendered depiction of the graft as it travels through the obturator foramen (*white arrows*) (Reproduced with kind permission from the Radiological Society of North America. Copyright 2008. Lopera J, Trimmer C, Josephs S, et al. Multidector CT angiography of infrainguinal arterial bypass. *Radiographics*. 2008;28:529–549.

femoral artery or profunda femoris alone are unusual and usually mycotic or traumatic.[324]

Femoral artery pseudoaneurysms may occur, especially in cases of trauma (invasive cardiac angiography or arterial reconstruction). The clinical course of femoral artery pseudoaneurysms is more ominous if left untreated.

Femoral artery aneurysms may be palpable or they may present with distal ischemia. In rare instances, they may rupture. The natural history of these aneurysms may be benign. However, a more malignant course may ensue if symptoms are present or if the aneurysm is large.

Femoral artery repair is certainly indicated if symptoms are present. However, there are no firm guidelines on when to repair asymptomatic femoral artery aneurysms because the natural history is not known with certainty. Also, no aneurysm size has been identified where the risk of rupture significantly increases or when complications rates increase. Most clinicians agree that if the patient is a good operative risk, true femoral artery aneurysms should be repaired when they are ≥ 2.5 cm. Smaller aneurysms or high-risk patients should be repaired if symptoms ensue or if significant enlargement occurs (0.5 cm in 1 year).[324]

Figures 8.34–8.36 demonstrate examples of femoral artery aneurysms. Figure 8.37 is an example of a femoral artery pseudoaneurysm.

8.2.3.3 Popliteal Artery Aneurysms

The popliteal artery is the most common site for development of a peripheral arterial aneurysm, accounting for 70% of all lower extremity arterial aneurysms. The estimated incidence of popliteal artery aneurysms is 0.1–2.8%.[322,324,325] They are 30 times more common in men than women.[325]

While the etiology of popliteal artery aneurysms is unclear, risks for development include hypertension, diabetes, smoking, and ischemic heart disease. The pathophysiology involves inflammatory infiltration with associated mediators such as matrix metalloproteinases that degrade the medial layer of the vessel wall.[325]

The identification of a popliteal artery aneurysm should prompt evaluation for aneurysms in the contralateral leg and in the aorta since they are bilateral in half of all cases and are associated with AAA in one-third of the cases.[326]

Sixty percent of popliteal aneurysms are symptomatic at presentation and 30% have limb threatening ischemia.[327,328]

As the popliteal artery aneurysm grows, it fills with thrombus. In fact, 40% of the time these aneurysms are discovered because of thrombosis or embolization.[329] Popliteal artery aneurysms ≥2 cm often contain large amounts of thrombus.[330] These aneurysms rarely present with rupture (2–4%).[330]

Intervention is indicated in aneurysms greater than 2 cm.[330-332] If mural thrombus is present, consideration may be given to correction at smaller sizes since the most common presentation is thrombosis, not rupture. The treatment for a

---→

FIGURE 8.27. (**a**) Depiction of volume-rendered reconstructions of a right axillary bifemoral bypass. Panel A demonstrates the highly calcified, tortuous native aorta (Ao). The bilateral iliac arteries (iliacs) are also highly calcified and severely diseased. The axillary bifemoral bypass graft (bypass) is marked by the triple arrow in panel A. The native femoral arteries distal to the graft are labeled "femorals." Panel B shows the proximal anastomosis of the axillary graft to the right axillary artery (*arrow head inside white circle*). This anastomosis is partially obscured by the high density contrast in the right subclavian vein crossing over the anastomosis. *Bypass* axillary bypass graft coursing caudally, *Axillary* right axillary artery, *RSC* right subclavian artery. Panel C demonstrates the distal anastomoses. The distal anastomosis of the axillary to right femoral bypass limb (AFB) is circled in white and the anastomosis of the axillary bypass graft to left femoral crossover limb (AFC) is within the white square. (**b**) Panels A, B, and C are depictions of the anastomoses of the bypass grafts in the patient from (a). Panel A is a multiplanar reformat (MPR) illustrating the axillary artery proximal anastomosis (*white circle*). MPR was necessary to limit the partial volume artifact from the calcium and venous contrast to permit visualization of the anastomosis. Panel B is a maximum intensity projection (MIP) showing the axillary bypass to right femoral anastomosis (*white arrow outlined in black*) and the proximal anastomosis of the axillary to left femoral crossover graft (*arrow head*). Panel C is an MIP demonstrating the distal anastomosis of the axillary to left femoral artery crossover graft (*white circle*). The native femoral artery (femoral) is seen moving from top to bottom and is heavily calcified. There is a tight stenosis in the native femoral artery just distal to the anastomosis (*arrow head*). Flow into the profunda artery (Pr) is uncompromised. *Crossover* Crossover graft.

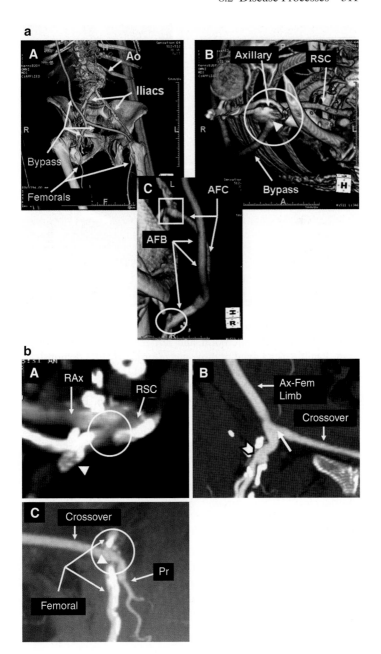

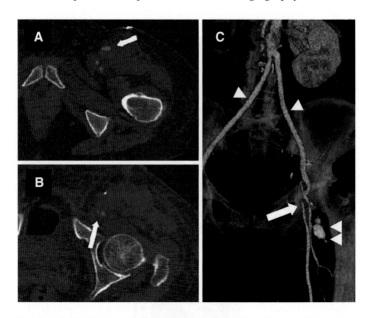

FIGURE 8.28. Demonstration of early bleeding in a patient who underwent an aorto-bifemoral and left femoral popliteal bypass graft. Panel A is an axial multiplanar reformat (MPR) demonstrating a large hematoma with dye extravasation (*arrow*). Panel B is an MPR just inferior to panel B demonstrating a partial thrombosis of the left femoral to popliteal bypass graft (*arrow*). Panel C is a volume-rendered, segmented, semitransparent reconstruction depicting the partial thrombosis of the left femoral to popliteal graft (*arrow*) and the dye extravasation (*double arrow head*). The aorto-bifemoral limbs appear intact (*single arrow heads*) (Reproduced with kind permission from the Radiological Society of North America. Copyright 2008. Lopera J, Trimmer C, Josephs S, et al. Multidector CT angiography of infrainguinal arterial bypass. *Radiographics*. 2008;28:529–549).

popliteal artery aneurysm is surgical correction or endovascular exclusion if possible. For endovascular therapy, the necessary arterial measurements include the diameter of the artery before and after the aneurysm, the length of the aneurysm, and the distance from the aneurysm to the branch vessels.

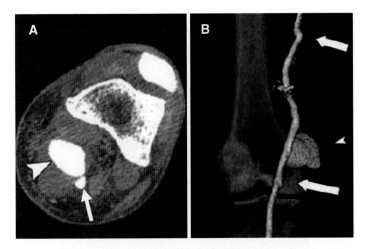

FIGURE 8.29. Demonstration of a late bleeding complication after a femoral to popliteal bypass graft surgery. The patient presented a few weeks after surgery with a painful, pulsatile mass. Panel A is an axial multiplanar reformat showing a large pseudoaneurysm (arrow head anterior to the graft [*arrow*]). Panel B shows the proximal and distal graft anastomoses (*arrows*) with the pseudoaneurysm in the middle of the graft (*arrow head*). The graft was infected and eventually replaced (Reproduced with kind permission from the Radiological Society of North America. Copyright 2008. Lopera J, Trimmer C, Josephs S, et al. Multidector CT angiography of infrainguinal arterial bypass. *Radiographics*. 2008;28:529–549.

Flexible stents such as the Gore Viabahn (Fig. 8.38) stent must be used to prevent stent fracture at the site of the knee. This endoprosthesis is constructed with a durable, reinforced, biocompatible, and expanded polytetrafluoroethylene (ePTFE, Teflon) liner attached to an external nitinol stent structure. The extreme flexibility of the Gore Viabahn enables it to better traverse tortuous areas of the aneurysm and conform more closely to the complex anatomy of the artery.

Most studies regarding the treatment of popliteal aneurysms are small case series. The 12- and 48-month follow-up show a primary patency rate for surgery versus endovascular repair of 100% versus 86.7% and 81.6% versus 80%, respectively.[333]

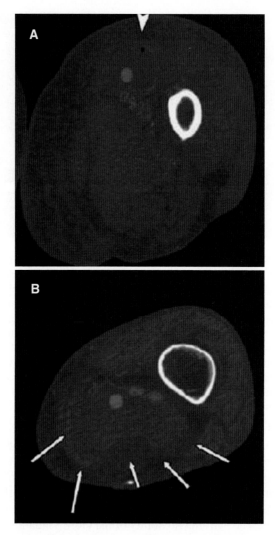

FIGURE 8.30. Panels A and B are maximum intensity projections of an infected femoral to popliteal bypass graft. A large fluid collection is noted around the lower extremity bypass graft (*arrows* in panel B). Air is seen within the fluid (*arrow head* in panel A) (Reproduced with kind permission from the Radiological Society of North America. Copyright 2008. Lopera J, Trimmer C, Josephs S, et al. Multidector CT angiography of infrainguinal arterial bypass. *Radiographics*. 2008;28:529–549).

TABLE 8.4. Classification system for popliteal entrapment syndrome proposed by Hai et al.

Type	Description
I	Normal medial head of gastrocnemius muscle. Popliteal artery is divided medially and has an aberrant course
II	Medial head of gastrocnemius muscle is located laterally. Normally coursing popliteal artery
III	Abnormal gastrocnemius muscle bundle surrounds a normally coursing popliteal artery
IV	Abnormal deep popliteal artery entrapped by the popliteus muscle or a fibrous band
V	Any type of entrapped popliteal artery that includes entrapment of the popliteal vein
VI	Normally positioned popliteal artery is entrapped by an anatomically normal but hypertrophied gastrocnemius muscle

Adapted from Hai Z, Guangrui S, Yuan Z, et al. CT angiography and MRI in patients with popliteal artery entrapment syndrome. *Am J Roentgenol.* 2008;191:1760–1766

Figures 8.39 and 8.40 demonstrate examples of popliteal artery aneurysms. Figure 8.41 demonstrates a successful stent exclusion of a popliteal artery aneurysm.

8.3 Accuracy of Peripheral Arterial CT Angiography

The main reason for imaging the lower extremities in patients with intermittent claudication, CLI, or ALI is to confirm the diagnosis of PAD and to identify an arterial lesion that is suitable for revascularization with either an endovascular or open surgical technique. In addition, alternative diagnoses may be identified. The current options for lower extremity imaging are invasive angiography, duplex ultrasound, magnetic resonance angiography (MRA), and CT angiography. Potential side effects and contraindications should be considered in choosing the imaging modality.

With the exception of duplex Doppler, all of these imaging options require a contrast medium that is potentially harmful. Iodinated contrast media required for invasive angiography and for CT angiography is potentially nephrotoxic. Gadolinium associated with MRA has been linked to nephrogenic systemic fibrosis. It should be noted, however, that invasive angiography may be performed with carbon dioxide to avoid nephrotoxicity.

While angiography has been the historic gold standard for evaluation of PAD, noninvasive angiography and CT angiography in particular can be a better imaging option. In particular, multidetector CT angiography has been widely adopted for the initial diagnostic evaluation and treatment-planning technique for PAD. Multislice CT enables fast imaging of the entire lower extremity and abdomen in one breath-hold at sub-millimeter isotropic voxel resolution. Advantages of CT angiography include a more complete and accurate assessment of the degree and characteristics of arterial calcification while adding incremental information regarding the length of chronic total occlusions since retrograde filling of distal segments is often more complete. In addition, access site planning may also be reliably performed with CT angiography.

Furthermore, CT techniques permit the ability to manipulate the images in three dimensions leading to improved eccentric stenosis detection and allowing evaluation of surrounding tissues which adds to the evaluation. Other

FIGURE 8.31. An example of popliteal entrapment syndrome in a young girl. Panel A shows a volume-rendered, segmented image with bone subtraction demonstrating a segmental occlusion at the level of the right popliteal artery with geniculate collateral development (*white oval* in panel A). Panel B is a maximum intensity projection showing a lateral location of the medial head of the gastrocnemius muscle (*long arrow*) and occlusion of the popliteal artery (*short arrow*). This is consistent with a type II anomaly (Table 8.4) (Reproduced with kind permission from the American Roentgen Ray Society. Copyright 2008. Hai Z, Guangrui S, Yan Z, et al. CT angiography and MRI in patients with popliteal artery entrapment syndrome. *Am J Roentgenol*. 2008;191:1760–1766.

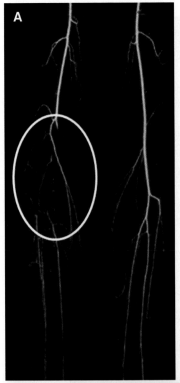

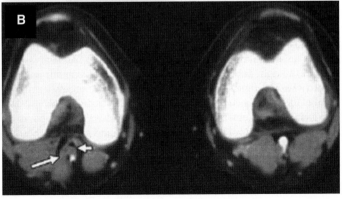

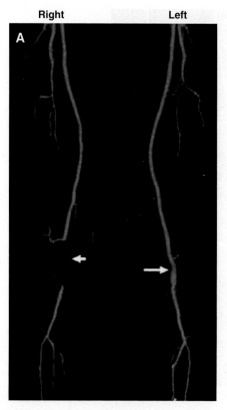

FIGURE 8.32. Bilateral popliteal entrapment in an older man shown in segmented, bone subtracted volume rendered recontructions (panel A). A type III anomaly is noted in the right knee and a type I anomaly is seen in the left knee (Table 8.4). Panels C and D are maximum intensity projections. The right leg demonstrates an aberrant accessory muscle band of the medial head of the right gastrocnemius muscle (*long arrow* in panel C) and an entrapped popliteal artery (*short arrow* in panel C). This anomaly has resulted in aneurysm formation and thrombosis of the right popliteal artery (*arrow* in panel B). Panel A demonstrates a volume-rendered image of the occluded right popliteal segment (*short arrow*). The left leg in panels B and C demonstrate an anatomically normal left gastrocnemius muscle but an aberrant left popliteal artery coursing medially resulting in a type I anomaly. The left popliteal artery (*long arrow* in panel A and *arrow heads* in panels B and C) is slightly aneurysmal (Reproduced with kind permission from the American Roentgen Ray Society. Copyright 2008. Hai Z, Guangrui S, Yan Z, et al. CT angiography and MRI in patients with popliteal artery entrapment syndrome. *Am J Roentgenol.* 2008;191:1760–1766).

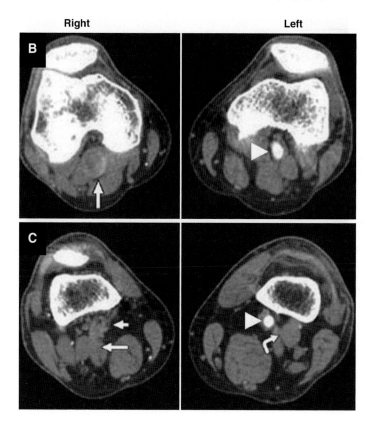

FIGURE 8.32. (continued).

advantages of CT angiography include its speed, convenience, and ability for cross-sectional imaging of the vessel. In addition, CT angiography (as well as MRA and Doppler) are noninvasive and are not associated with the risks of an invasive procedure such as direct arteriography.

Unique limitations of CT include the blooming artifact caused by the presence of calcium and by stents. These artifacts can preclude accurate luminal assessment particularly in smaller vessels. Doppler is advantageous because of its ability to assess blood flow. Ultimately, the final choice in diagnostic imaging technique and revascularization planning strategy depends on physician and institutional preference and the expertise of the treating physician and institution.

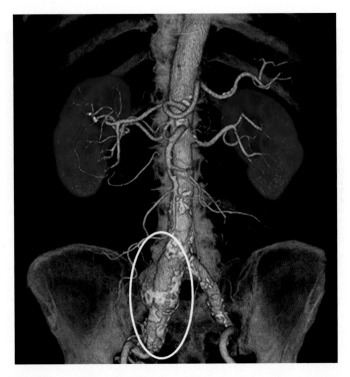

FIGURE 8.33. A volume-rendered, segmented, semitransparent recon-struction of an extensive right iliac artery aneurysm (*white oval*).

Although prospectively designed studies with CT angiog-raphy are currently lacking, there are emerging data that the sensitivity, specificity, and accuracy of this technique may rival invasive angiography.[336,337] The accuracy of lower extremity CT angiography has been reported to be quite good. Sensitivity for stenoses ≥50% range for 89–100% and specificities range from 92% to 100%.[338,339,340,341,342] No difference in diagnostic accuracy has been found for CT angiography of the suprapo-pliteal region versus the infrapopliteal region.[343] Sensitivities of 100% have been documented for CT angiography in diag-nosing femoral artery occlusion, popliteal occlusion, and occlusion of the tibial-peroneal trunk.[335,336,337] There are reports

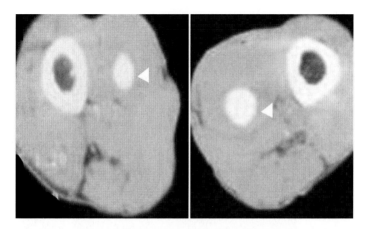

FIGURE 8.34. A maximum intensity projection image demonstrating bilateral superficial femoral artery aneurysms (*white arrow heads*).

of sensitivities in the 94% range for CT angiographic identification of tibial artery occlusions.[335, 336, 337] In addition, the specificities for femoral, popliteal, and tibial-peroneal trunk occlusions are 100%, 99% and 98%, respectively.[335,336,337] In addition, CT angiography has been shown to be very sensitive and accurate in diagnosing popliteal artery aneurysms. In one study, CT angiography was diagnostic in all cases and all complications of the aneurysm were identified.[338]

For grading of high-grade stenoses (75–99%), the sensitivities are 88% and 73%, respectively for the superficial femoral artery and the popliteal artery including the tibial-peroneal trunk. The specificities are 94% and 100%, respectively.[344] CT angiography may be difficult in these locations due to the frequency, severity, and diffuse nature of heavily calcified atherosclerosis. Magnetic resonance angiography (MRA) may be more reliable in these regions or when calcific disease is known or suspected.

The sensitivity and specificity between CT angiography, duplex ultrasound and digital subtraction angiography are equal for the evaluation of peripheral arterial bypass grafts. Sensitivities and specificities are reported to be in the 91–100% range.[345, 346]

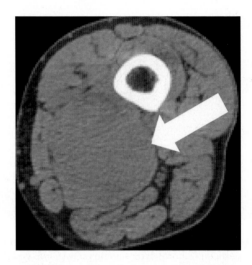

FIGURE 8.35. Illustration of a non-contrasted axial image of a very large superficial femoral artery aneurysm (*large white arrow*).

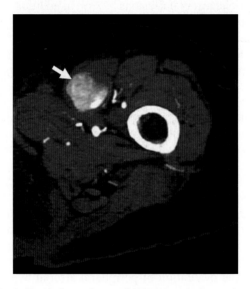

FIGURE 8.36. Depiction of a multiplanar reformat of a partially thrombosed superficial femoral artery aneurysm (*white arrow*).

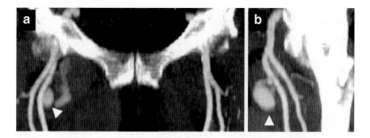

FIGURE 8.37. An example of a femoral artery pseudoaneurysm (*white arrow head in panels A and B*). Panel A is an anterior thick maximum intensity projection (MIP) and panel B is a lateral MIP.

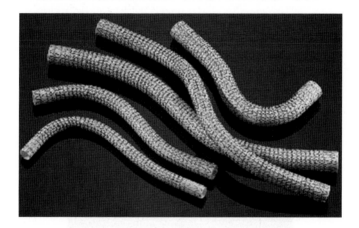

FIGURE 8.38. Gore Viabahn stent (WL Gore and Associates, Flagstaff, Arizona) (Reproduced with kind permission from HMP Communications. Copyright 2005. Schussler J and Johnson K. Exclusion of a Renal Artery Aneurysm with a Viabahn Self-expanding Covered Stent. Vascular Disease Management. 2005;2(3)).

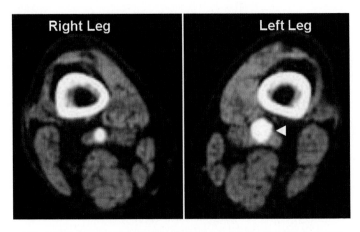

FIGURE 8.39. Demonstration of an axial multiplanar reformat of a left popliteal artery aneurysm (*white arrow head*).

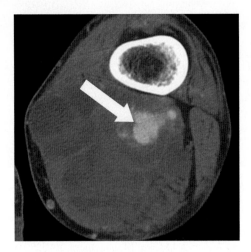

FIGURE 8.40. A multiplanar reformat of a large partially thrombosed popliteal artery aneurysm (*white arrow*). There is partial extrusion of dye into the soft tissue from this aneurysm.

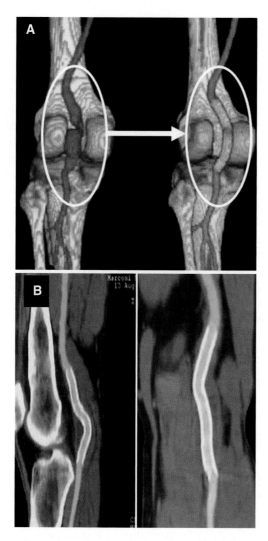

FIGURE 8.41. An example of a successful stent exclusion of a popliteal artery aneurysm. Panel A is a volume-rendered, segmented reconstruction demonstrating the aneurysm (*inside left white oval* in panel A) before stenting and after stenting (*inside right white oval* in panel A). Panel B is a maximum intensity projection of the successful popliteal stent (Reproduced with kind permission from HMP Communications. Copyright 2007. Ghotbi R, Sotiriou A, Schonhofer S, et al. Stent-graft placement in popliteal artery aneurysms: midterm results. *Vasc Dis Manag.* 2007;4(4)).

8.4 Approach to Reading Peripheral Arterial CT Angiography

As is customary for all CT angiography evaluations, a systematic approach is recommended to avoid omissions. First, the quality of the study and the contrast adequacy and timing are assessed. Next, an overall anatomical overview is obtained using the three-dimensional volume-rendered images. Areas of concern are identified, stents and bypass grafts are located if present, clues to aneurysm formation are obtained, calcified areas may be located, and anatomic relationships may be characterized.

Ultimately, however, the work horse reconstruction technique for assessing the lower extremity arterial circulation is the maximum intensity projection (MIP) axial images. The arterial anatomy is followed by first evaluating the proximal most vessels and subsequently moving to the more distal vessels, one segment at a time and one leg at a time. We recommend completely analyzing each limb, individually. Sagittal and oblique views are employed when necessary to evaluate more complicated anatomy and multiplanar (MPR) reconstructions and curved multiplanar (cMPR) techniques are utilized when needed to confirm diagnoses and better characterize the atherosclerotic burden.

The extent, location, and severity of any atherosclerosis must be identified and documented. Calcification must be characterized and subjectively quantified. Be aware of collaterals in odd or unusual locations that may provide clues to pathology.

Occlusions should be noted and appropriately characterized. It is important to describe the entry point of the occlusion site. For example, describing the angle of the entry point may help with choice of access site. In addition, noting whether the entry point has a "nipple" or is simply a stump may help to delineate the chance for procedural success (crossing of the guidewire). It may also aid in choosing the appropriate equipment since a "nipple" appearance suggests an entry point for the wire.

The presence of collaterals at the entry point should be noted. The presence of collaterals makes the procedure more challenging and reduces the chance for success since the wire will preferentially travel through collateral rather than through an occlusion point. The location and distribution of calcium in and adjacent to the occluded territory is also very helpful. Aneurysms should be excluded. If present, comment on the location, size, and any associated thrombus.

Dissections should also be characterized and documented if present. The location, extent, and branch vessel involvement should be noted. Comment on ancillary findings if present.

For bypass grafts, multiple questions must be answered. Are the proximal and distal anastomoses patent? Are the inflow and run-off vessels patent and adequate? Have any kinks or in-graft stenoses been identified? Are there any findings suggestive of graft infection or bleeding? Have any fistulas been identified? Are any ancillary findings present?

In addition, peripheral CT angiography is important for procedural planning. It may help in choosing the most appropriate procedural technique by characterizing the access site for various devices, by sizing the vessel, and by determining the stenosis characteristics, calcifications, eccentricity, and length.

Finally, standardized reporting should be concise, organized, and clinically relevant.

References

1. Pelberg R, Mazur W. *Cardiac CT Angiography Manual*. London: Springer; 2007. Ref. type: serial (book, monograph).
2. Halliday AW, Thomas DJ, Mansfield AO. The asymptomatic carotid surgery trial (ACST). *Int Angiol*. 1995;14(1):18–20.
3. Toole JF. ACAS recommendations for carotid endarterectomy. ACAS executive committee. *Lancet*. 1996;347(8994):121.
4. Eliasziw M et al. North American Symptomatic Carotid Endarterectomy Trial. Significance of plaque ulceration in symptomatic patients with high-grade carotid stenosis. *Stroke*. 1994;25:304–308.
5. Qureshi AI et al. Guidelines for screening of extracranial carotid artery disease: a statement for healthcare professionals from the multidisciplinary practice guidelines committee of the American Society of Neuroimaging; cosponsored by the Society of Vascular and Interventional Neurology. *J Neuroimaging*. 2007;17:19–47.
6. Biller J et al. Guidelines for carotid endarterectomy. A statement for healthcare professionals from a special writing group of the stroke council, American Heart Association. *Circulation*. 1998;97:501–509.
7. Roubin GS, New G, Iyer SS et al. Immediate and late clinical outcomes of carotid artery stenting in patients with symptomatic and asymptomatic carotid artery stenosis: a 5-year prospective analysis. *Circulation*. 2001;103(4):532–537.

DOI: 10.1007/978-1-84996-260-5_References,
© Springer-Verlag London Limited 2011

8. Sheon RP, Moskowitz RW, Goldberg VM. *Soft Tissue Rheumatic Pain: Recognition, Management, Prevention.* 3rd ed. Baltimore: Williams & Wilkins; 1996.

9. Dale WA, Lewis MR. Management of thoracic outlet syndrome. *Ann Surg.* 1975;181:575.

10. Conn J Jr. Thoracic outlet syndromes. *Surg Clin N Am.* 1974; 54:155.

11. Roos DB. Congenital anomalies associated with thoracic outlet syndrome. *Am J Surg.* 1976;132:771.

12. McGough EC, Pearce MB, Byrne JP. Management of thoracic outlet syndrome. *J Thorac Cardiov Sur.* 1979;77:169. Tyson RR, Kaplan GF. Modern concepts of diagnosis and treatment of the thoracic outlet syndrome. *Orthop Clin N Am.* 1975;6:507.

13. Novak CB, Collins ED, Mackinnon SE. Outcome following conservative management of thoracic outlet syndrome. *J Hand Surg.* 1995;20:542.

14. Donaghy M, Matkovic Z, Morris P. Surgery for suspected neurogenic thoracic outlet syndrome: a follow up study. *J Neurol Neurosurg Psychiatry.* 1999;67:602.

15. Wigley FM. Clinical practice. Raynaud's phenomenon. *N Engl J Med.* 2002;347:1001.

16. Maricq HR, Carpentier PH, Weinrich MC, et al. Geographic variation in the prevalence of Raynaud's phenomenon: Charleston, SC, USA, vs Tarentaise, Savoie, France. *J Rheumatol.* 1993;20:70.

17. Gelber AC, Wigley FM, Stallings RY, et al. Symptoms of Raynaud's phenomenon in an inner-city African-American community: prevalence and self-reported cardiovascular comorbidity. *J Clin Epidemiol.* 1999;52:441.

18. Brennan P, Silman A, Black C, et al. Validity and reliability of three methods used in the diagnosis of Raynaud's phenomenon. *Br J Rheumatol.* 1993;32:357.

19. Olin JW. Thromboangiitis obliterans (Buerger's disease). *N Engl J Med.* 2000;342:864.

20. Lie JT. The rise and fall and resurgence of thromboangiitis obliterans (Buerger's disease). *Acta Pathol Jpn.* 1989;39:153.

21. Mills JL, Taylor LM, Porter JM. Buerger's disease in the modern era. *Am J Surg.* 1987;154:123.

22. Mills JL, Porter JM. Buerger's disease (thromboangiitis obliterans). *Ann Vasc Surg*. 1991;5:570.
23. Lie JT. Diagnosic histopathology of major systemic and pulmonary vasculitic syndromes. *Rheum Dis Clin N Am*. 1990;16:269.
24. Olin JW. Thromboangiitis obliterans (Buerger's disease). *N Engl J Med*. 2000;342:864.
25. Shionoya S. Diagnostic criteria of Buerger's disease. *Int J Cardiol*. 1998;66(suppl 1):S243.
26. Randoux B et al. Carotid artery stenosis: prospective comparison of CT, three-dimensional gadolinium-enhanced MR, and conventional angiography. *Radiology*. 2001;220:179–185.
27. Bartlett ES, Walers SP et al. Quantification of carotid stenosis on CT angiography. *Am J Neuroradiol*. 2006;27:13–19.
28. Bickerstaff LK et al. Thoracic aortic aneurysms: a population-based study. *Surgery*. 1982;92(6):1103–1108.
29. Crawford ES, Cohen ES. Aortic aneurysm: a multifocal disease. Presidential address. *Arch Surg*. 1982;117(11):1393–1400. Pressler V, McNamara JJ. Aneurysm of the thoracic aorta. Review of 260 cases. *J Thorac Cardiov Sur*. 1985;89(1):50–54.
30. Isselbacher EM. Thoracic and abdominal aortic aneurysms. *Circulation*. 2005;111(6):816–828.
31. Abbara S, Kalva S, Cury RC et al. Thoracic aortic disease: spectrum of multidetector computed tomography imaging findings. *J Cardiovasc Comput Tomogr*. 2007;1(1):40–54.
32. Reed et al. Are aortic aneurysms caused by atherosclerosis? *Circulation*. 1992;85(1):205–211.
33. Tilson MD. Aortic aneurysms and atherosclerosis (editorial). *Circulation*. 1992;85:378.
34. MacSweeney ST et al. Pathogenesis of abdominal aortic aneurysm. *Br J Surg*. 1994;81(7):935–941.
35. Adams JN, Trent RJ. Aortic complications of Marfan's syndrome. *Lancet*. 1998;352(9142):1722–1723.
36. Kornbluth M et al. Clinical outcome in the Marfan syndrome with ascending aortic dilatation followed annually by echocardiography. *Am J Cardiol*. 1999;84(6):753–755. A9.
37. Lung B, Gohlke-Barwolf C, Tornos P et al. Recommendations on the management of the asymptomatic patient with valvular heart disease. *Eur Heart J*. 2002;23:1252.

38. Bruno L et al. Cardiac, skeletal, and ocular abnormalities in patients with Marfan's syndrome and in their relatives. Comparison with the cardiac abnormalities in patients with kyphoscoliosis. *Br Heart J*. 1984;51(2):220–230.

39. Coady MA et al. Familial patterns of thoracic aortic aneurysms. *Arch Surg*. 1999;134(4):361–367.

40. Pannu H et al. Mutations in transforming growth factor-beta receptor type II cause familial thoracic aortic aneurysms and dissections. *Circulation*. 2005;112(4):513–520.

41. Crawford SE et al. Thoracoabdominal aortic aneurysms: preoperative and intraoperative factors determining immediate and long term results of operations in 605 patients. *J Vasc Surg*. 1986;3:389–404.

42. Griepp RB et al. The natural history of thoracic aortic aneurysm. *Semin Thorac Cardiovasc Surg*. 1991;3(4):258–265.

43. Clouse WD et al. Improved prognosis of thoracic aortic aneurysms: a population-based study. *JAMA*. 1998;280(22): 1926–1929.

44. Juvonen T et al. Prospective study of the natural history of thoracic aortic aneurysm. *Ann Thorac Surg*. 1997;63(6): 1533–1545.

45. Coady MA et al. Surgical intervention criteria for thoracic aortic aneurysms: a study of growth rates and complications. *Ann Thorac Surg*. 1999;67(6):1922–1926.

46. Bonser RS et al. Clinical and patho-anatomical factors affecting expansion of thoracic aortic aneurysms. *Heart*. 2000;84(3): 277–283.

47. Dapunt OE et al. The natural history of thoracic aortic aneurysms. *J Thorac Cardiovasc Surg*. 1994;107(5):1323–1332.

48. Davies RR et al. Yearly rupture or dissection rates for thoracic aortic aneurysms: simple prediction based on size. *Ann Thorac Surg*. 2002;73(1):17–27.

49. Coady MA, Rizzo JA, Hammond GL et al. Surgical intervention criteria for thoracic aortic aneurysms: A study of growth rates and complications. *Ann Thorac Surg*. 1999;67:1922.

50. Elefteriades JA. Natural history of thoracic aortic aneurysms: indications for surgery, and surgical versus nonsurgical risks. *Ann Thorac Surg*. 2002;74:S1877.

51. Lobato AC, Puech-Leao P. Predictive factors for rupture of thoracoabdominal aortic aneurysm. *J Vasc Surg*. 1998;27:446.

52. Bonow RO, Carabello BA, Chatterjee K et al. ACC/AHA 2006 guidelines for the management of patients with valvular heart disease. A report of the American College of Cardiology/ American Heart Association Task Force on practice guidelines (writing committee to revise the 1998 guidelines for the management of patients with valvular heart disease). *J Am Coll Cardiol*. 2006;48:e1.

53. Gott VL et al. Surgical treatment of aneurysm of the ascending aorta in the Marfan syndrome. Results of composite-graft repair in 50 patients. *N Engl J Med*. 1986;314(17): 1070–1074.

54. Ergin MA et al. Surgical treatment of the dilated ascending aorta: when and how. *Ann Thorac Surg*. 1999;67(6):1834–1839.

55. Ehrlich M et al. Endovascular stent graft repair for aneurysms on the descending thoracic aorta. *Ann Thorac Surg*. 1998;66(1): 19–24.

56. Semba CP et al. Thoracic aortic aneurysm repair with endovascular stent-grafts. *Vasc Med*. 1997;2(2):98–103.

57. Dake MD et al. The "first generation" of endovascular stent-grafts for patients with aneurysms of the descending thoracic aorta. *J Thorac Cardiovasc Surg*. 1998;116(5):689–703.

58. Grabenwoger M et al. Thoracic aortic aneurysms: treatment with endovascular self-expandable stent grafts. *Ann Thorac Surg*. 2000;69(2):441–445.

59. Doss M et al. Emergency endovascular interventions for acute thoracic aortic rupture: four-year follow-up. *J Thorac Cardiovasc Surg*. 2005;129(3):645–651.

60. Leurs LJ et al. Endovascular treatment of thoracic aortic diseases: combined experience from the EUROSTAR and United Kingdom Thoracic Endograft registries. *J Vasc Surg*. 2004; 40(4):670–679.

61. Katzen BT et al. Endovascular repair of abdominal and thoracic aortic aneurysms. *Circulation*. 2005;112(11):1663–1675.

62. Appoo JJ et al. Thoracic aortic stent grafting: improving results with newer generation investigational devices. *J Thorac Cardiovasc Surg*. 2006;131(5):1087–1094.

63. Demers P, Miller DC, Mitchell RS et al. Midterm results of endovascular repair of descending thoracic aortic aneurysms with first-generation stent grafts. *J Thorac Cardiovasc Surg.* 2004;127:664.

64. Svensson LG et al. Experience with 1509 patients undergoing thoracoabdominal aortic operations. *J Vasc Surg.* 1993;17(2):357–368; discussion 368–370.

65. Bavarua JE et al. Retrograde cerebral and distal aortic perfusion during ascending and thoracoabdominal aortic operations. *Ann Thorac Surg.* 1995;60(2):345–352.

66. Jacobs MJ et al. Reduced renal failure following thoracoabdominal aortic aneurysm repair by selective perfusion. *Eur J Cardiothorac Surg.* 1998;14(2):201–205.

67. Hollier LH et al. Risk of spinal cord dysfunction in patients undergoing thoracoabdominal aortic replacement. *Am J Surg.* 1992;164(3):210–213; discussion 213–214.

68. Shapira OM et al. Improved clinical outcomes after operation of the proximal aorta: a 10-year experience. *Ann Thorac Surg.* 1999;67(4):1030–1037.

69. LeMaire SA et al. A new predictive model for adverse outcomes after elective thoracoabdominal aortic aneurysm repair. *Ann Thorac Surg.* 2001;71(4):1233–1238.

70. Mastroroberto P, Chello M. Emergency thoracoabdominal aortic aneurysm repair: clinical outcome. *J Thorac Cardiov Sur.* 1999;118(3):477–481; discussion 481–482.

71. Schepens MA et al. Reoperations on the ascending aorta and aortic root: pitfalls and results in 134 patients. *Ann Thorac Surg.* 1999;68(5):1676–1680.

72. Mukherjee D, Evangelista A, Nienaber CA et al. Implications of periaortic hematoma in patients with acute aortic dissection (from the International Registry of Acute Aortic Dissection). *Am J Cardiol.* 2005;96:1734.

73. Bickerstaff LK, Pairolero PC, Hollier LH. Thoracic aortic aneurysms: a population-based study. *Surgery.* 1982;92:1103.

74. Meszaros I, Morocz J, Szlavi J et al. Epidemiology and clinicopathology of aortic dissection. *Chest.* 2000;117:1271.

75. Clouse WD, Hallett JW Jr, Schaff HV et al. Acute aortic dissection: population-based incidence compared with degenerative aortic aneurysm rupture. *Mayo Clin Proc.* 2004;79:176.

76. Sorenson HR, Olsen H. Ruptured and dissecting aneurysms of the aorta. Incidents and prospects of surgery. *Acta Chir Scand.* 1964;128:644–650.

77. Larson EW, Edwards WD. Risk factors for aortic dissection: A necropsy study of 161 cases. *Am J Cardiol.* 1984;53:849.

78. Chavanon O, Carrier M, Cartier R et al. Increased incidence of acute ascending aortic dissection with off-pump aortocoronary bypass surgery? *Ann Thorac Surg.* 2001;71:117.

79. Nienaber CA, Fattori R, Mehta RH et al. Gender-related differences in acute aortic dissection. *Circulation.* 2004;109:3014.

80. Hagan PG, Nienaber CA, Isselbacher EM et al. The International Registry of Acute Aortic Dissection (IRAD): new insights into an old disease. *JAMA.* 2000;283:897.

81. Hagl C, Ergin MA, Galla JD et al. Delayed chronic type A dissection following CABG: implications for evolving techniques of revascularization. *J Card Surg.* 2000;15:362.

82. Svensson LG et al. Intimal tear without hematoma: An important variant of aortic dissection that can elude current imaging techniques. *Circulation.* 1999;99:1331.

83. Roberts CS, Roberts WC. Dissection of the aorta associated with congenital malformation of the aortic valve. *J Am Coll Cardiol.* 1991;17:712.

84. Nistri S, Sorbo MD, Marin M et al. Aortic root dilatation in young men with normally functioning bicuspid aortic valves. *Heart.* 1999;82:19.

85. Hahn RT, Roman MJ, Mogtader AH, Devereux RB. Association of aortic dilatation with regurgitant, stenotic and functionally normal bicuspid aortic valves. *J Am Coll Cardiol.* 1992;19:283.

86. Lin AE, Lippe B, Rosenfeld RG. Further delineation of aortic dilation, dissection, and rupture in patients with Turner syndrome. *Pediatrics.* 1998;102:e12.

87. Januzzi JL, Isselbacher EM, Fattori R et al. Characterizing the young patient with aortic dissection: results from the International Registry of Aortic Dissection (IRAD). *J Am Coll Cardiol.* 2004;43:665.

88. Spittell PC, Spittell JA Jr, Joyce JW et al. Clinical features and differential diagnosis of aortic dissection: Experience with 236 cases (1980 through 1990). *Mayo Clin Proc.* 1993;68:642.

89. Hagan PG, Nienaber CA, Isselbacher EM et al. The International Registry of Acute Aortic Dissection (IRAD): new insights into an old disease. *JAMA*. 2000;283:897.

90. Smith MD, Cassidy JM, Souther S et al. Transesophageal echocardiography in the diagnosis of traumatic rupture of the aorta. *N Engl J Med*. 1995;332:356.

91. Elefteriades JA, Hatzaras I, Tranquilli MA et al. Weight lifting and rupture of silent aortic aneurysms. *JAMA*. 2003; 290:2803.

92. Nienaber CA, Fattori R, Mehta RH et al. Gender-related differences in acute aortic dissection. *Circulation*. 2004; 109:3014.

93. Bossone E, Rampoldi V, Nienaber CA et al. Usefulness of pulse deficit to predict in-hospital complications and mortality in patients with acute type A aortic dissection. *Am J Cardiol*. 2002;89:851.

94. Nienaber CA, Eagle KA. Aortic dissection: new frontiers in diagnosis and management: part I: from etiology to diagnostic strategies. *Circulation*. 2003;108:628.

95. Nallamothu BK, Mehta RH, Saint S et al. Syncope in acute aortic dissection. Diagnostic, prognostic, and clinical implications. *Am J Med*. 2002;113:468.

96. Park SW, Hutchison S, Mehta RH et al. Association of painless acute aortic dissection with increased mortality. *Mayo Clin Proc*. 2004;79:1252.

97. Tsai TT, Nienaber CA, Eagle KA. Acute aortic syndromes. *Circulation*. 2005;112:3802.

98. Daily PO, Trueblood HW, Stinson EB et al. Management of acute aortic dissections. *Ann Thorac Surg*. 1970;10:237.

99. Debakey ME, Henly WS, Cooley DA et al. Surgical management of dissecting aneurysm of the aorta. *J Thorac Cardiovasc Surg*. 1965;49:130–149.

100. Daily PO, Trueblood HW, Stinson EB et al. Management of acute aortic dissections. *Ann Thorac Surg*. 1970;10: 237–247.

101. Miller DC, Mitchell RS, Oyer PE et al. Independent detriments of operative mortality for patients with aortic dissections. *Circulation*. 1984;70:153–164.

102. Miller DC. The continuing dilemma concerning medical versus surgical management of patients with acute type B dissections. *Semin Thorac Cardiovasc Surg.* 1993;5:33–46.

103. Doss M, Wood JP, Balzer J et al. Emergency endovascular interventions for acute thoracic aortic rupture: four-year follow-up. *J Thorac Cardiovasc Surg.* 2005;129:645.

104. Lauterbach SR, Cambria RP, Brewster DC et al. Contemporary management of aortic branch compromise resulting from acute aortic dissection. *J Vasc Surg.* 2001;33:1185–1192.

105. Beregi JP, Prat A, Gaxotte V et al. Endovascular treatment for dissection of the descending aorta. *Lancet.* 2000;356: 482–483.

106. Panneton JM, The SH, Cherry KJ et al. Aortic fenestration for acute or chronic aortic dissection: an uncommon but effective procedure. *J Vasc Surg.* 2000;32:711–721.

107. Gaxotte V, Cocheteux B, Haulon S. Relationship of intimal flap position to endovascular treatment of malperfusion syndromes in aortic dissection. *J Endovasc Ther.* 2003;10:719–727.

108. Davies M, Guest PJ. Developmental abnormalities of the great vessels of the thorax and their embryologic basis. *Br J Radiol.* 2003;76:491–502.

109. Smetana GW, Shmerling RH. Does this patient have temporal arteritis? *JAMA.* 2002;287(1):92–101.

110. Lawrence RC et al. Estimates of the prevalence of arthritis and selected musculoskeletal disorders in the United States. *Arthritis Rheum.* 1998;41(5):778–799.

111. Hunder GG et al. The American College of Rheumatology 1990 criteria for the classification of giant cell arteritis. *Arthritis Rheum.* 1990;33(8):1122–1128.

112. Evans JM et al. Thoracic aortic aneurysm and rupture in giant cell arteritis. A descriptive study of 41 cases. *Arthritis Rheum.* 1994;37(10):1539–1547.

113. Klein RG et al. Large artery involvement in giant cell (temporal) arteritis. *Ann Intern Med.* 1975;83(6):806–812.

114. Nuenninghoff DM et al. Incidence and predictors of large-artery complications (aortic aneurysm, aortic dissection, and/or large-artery stenosis) in patients with giant cell arteritis: a population-based study over 50 years. *Arthritis Rheum.* 2003;48(12):3522–3531.

115. Liozon E et al. Silent, or masked, giant cell arteritis is associated with a strong inflammatory response and a benign short term course. *J Rheumatol*. 2003;30(6):1272–1276.

116. Gonzalez-Gay MA et al. Giant cell arteritis: disease patterns of clinical presentation in a series of 240 patients. *Medicine (Baltimore)*. 2005;84(5):269–276.

117. Miller NR. Visual manifestations of temporal arteritis. *Rheum Dis Clin N Am*. 2001;27(4):781–797.

118. Klein RG et al. Large artery involvement in giant cell (temporal) arteritis. *Ann Intern Med*. 1975;83(6):806–812.

119. Ninet JP et al. Subclavian and axillary involvement in temporal arteritis and polymyalgia rheumatica. *Am J Med*. 1990; 88(1):13–20.

120. Salvarani C et al. Giant cell arteritis: involvement of intracranial arteries. *Arthritis Rheum*. 2006;55(6):985–989.

121. Koide K. Takayasu arteritis in Japan. *Heart Vessels Suppl*. 1992;7:48–54.

122. Lupi-Herrera E et al. Takayasu's arteritis. Clinical study of 107 cases. *Am Heart J*. 1977;93(1):94–103.

123. Arend WP et al. The American College of Rheumatology 1990 criteria for the classification of Takayasu arteritis. *Arthritis Rheum*. 1990;33(8):1129–1134.

124. Hata A et al. Angiographic findings of Takayasu arteritis: new classification. *Int J Cardiol*. 1996;54(Suppl):S155–S163.

125. Cid MC et al. Large vessel vasculitides. *Curr Opin Rheumatol*. 1998;10(1):18–28.

126. Sharma BK, Jain S, Sagar S. Systemic manifestations of Takayasu arteritis: the expanding spectrum. *Int J Cardiol*. 1997;54(Suppl):S149–S154.

127. Tsutsumi M et al. Aberrant right subclavian artery – three case reports. *Neurol Med Chir*. (Tokyo) 2002;42:396–398.

128. Davies M, Guest PJ. Developmental abnormalities of the great vessels of the thorax and their embryologic basis. *Br J Radiol*. 2004;76:491–502.

129. Gray H. *The Anatomy of the Human Body*. 20th ed. Thoroughly revised and re-edited by Lewis WH. Philadelphia: Lea & Febiger; 1918. New York: Bartleby.com; 2000.

130. Powell AJ et al. Vascular rings and slings. In: Kean JF, Lock JE, Fyler DC, eds. *Nadas' Pediatric Cardiology*. 2nd ed. Philadelphia: Saunders Elsevier; 2006:811.

131. Humphrey C et al. Decade of experience with vascular rings at a single institution. *Pediatrics*. 2006;177:e903.

132. Turner A et al. Vascular rings-presentation, investigation and outcome. *Eur J Pediatr*. 2005;164:266.

133. Van Son J, Konstantinov I, Burckhard F. Kommerell and Kommerell's Diverticulum. *Tex Heart Inst J*. 2002;29(2): 109–112.

134. Erbel R, Engberding R, Daniel W et al. Echocardiography in diagnosis of aortic dissection. *Lancet*. 1989;1:457.

135. Nienaber CA, von Kodolitsch Y, Nicolas V et al. The diagnosis of thoracic aortic dissection by noninvasive imaging procedures. *N Engl J Med*. 1993;328:1.

136. Sommer T, Fehske W, Holzknecht N et al. Aortic dissection: a comparative study of diagnosis with spiral CT, multiplanar transesophageal echocardiography, and MR imaging. *Radiology*. 1996;199:347.

137. Sebastia C, Pallisa E, Quiroga S et al. Aortic dissection: diagnosis and follow-up with helical CT. *Radiographics*. 1999;19:45.

138. Hamada S, Takamiya M, Kimura K et al. Type A aortic dissection: Evaluation with ultrafast CT. *Radiology*. 1992;183:155.

139. Hayter RG, Rhea JT, Small A et al. Suspected aortic dissection and other aortic disorders: multi-detector row CT in 373 cases in the emergency setting. *Radiology*. 2006;238:841.

140. Loubeyre P, Angelie E, Grozel F et al. Spiral CT artifact that simulates aortic dissection: image reconstruction with use of 180° and 360° linear-interpolation algorithms. *Radiology*. 1997;205:153.

141. Schertler T, Glucker T, Wildermuth S et al. Comparison of retrospectively ECG-gated and nongated MDCT of the chest in an emergency setting regarding workflow, image quality, and diagnostic certainty. *Emerg Radiol*. 2005;12:19.

142. Vasile N, Mathieu D, Keita K et al. Computed tomography of thoracic aortic dissection: accuracy and pitfalls. *J Comput Assist Tomogr*. 1986;10:211.

143. Pande RL, Beckman JA. Abdominal aortic aneurysm: populations at risk and how to screen. *J Vasc Interv Radiol*. 2008;19:S2–S8.

144. Ashton HA, Buxton MJ, Day NE et al. The multicenter aneurysm screening study (MASS) into the effect of abdominal

aortic aneurysm screening in men: a randomized controlled trial. *Lancet*. 2002;360:1531–1539.

145. Norman PE, Jamrozik K, Lawrence-Brown MM et al. Population based randomized controlled trial on impact of screening on mortality from abdominal aortic aneurysm. *Br Med J*. 2004;329:1259.

146. Bengtsson H, Sonesson B, Bergqvist D. Incidence and prevalence of abdominal aortic aneurysm, estimated by necropsy studies and population screening by ultrasound. *Ann N Y Acad Sci*. 1996;800:1–24.

147. Lederle FA, Johnson GR, Wilson SE et al. The aneurysm detection and management study screening program: Validation cohort and final results. aneurysm detection and management Veterans Affairs Cooperative Study Investigators. *Arch Intern Med*. 2000;160:1425–1430.

148. Rasmussen TE, Hallett JW Jr. Inflammatory aortic aneurysms: a clinical review with new perspectives in pathogenesis. *Ann Surg*. 1997;225:155–164.

149. Pennell RC, Hollier LH, Lie JT et al. Inflammatory abdominal aortic aneurysms: a thirty-year review. *J Vasc Surg*. 1985;2:859–869.

150. U.S. Preventive Services Task Force. Screening for abdominal aortic aneurysm: recommendation statement. *Ann Intern Med*. 2005;142:198–2002.

151. Upchurch GR Jr. et al. Abdominal aortic aneurysm. *Am Fam Physician*. 2006;73(7):303–310.

152. Siegel CL et al. Abdominal aortic aneurysm morphology: CT features in patients with ruptured and nonruptured aneurysms. *Am J Roentgenol*. 1994;163(5):1123–1129.

153. U.S. Preventive Services Task Force. Screening for abdominal aortic aneurysm: recommendation statement. *Ann Intern Med*. 2005;142:198–2002.

154. Gonsalves CF. The hyperattenuating crescent sign. *Radiology*. 1999;211:37–38.

155. Thammaroj J et al. Predictive CT features in ruptured abdominal aortic aneurysm. *J Med Assoc Thai*. 2006;89(4): 434–40.

156. Kent KC et al. Screening for abdominal aortic aneurysm: a consensus statement. *J Vasc Surg*. 2004;39:267–269.

157. Creager MA, Loscalzo J and Dzau VJ. *Vascular Medicine: A Companion to Braunwald's Heart Disease*. Philadelphia: Elsevier; 2006:543–606.
158. Lederle FA, Leimel DL. The rational clinical examination. Does this patient have abdominal aortic aneurysm? *JAMA*. 1999;281:77–82.
159. Giannoglou G et al. Predicting the risk of rupture of abdominal aortic aneurysms by utilizing various geometrical parameters: revisiting the diameter criterion. *Angiology*. 2006; 57(4):487–494.
160. Fillinger M. The long-term relationship of wall stress to the natural history of abdominal aortic aneurysms (finite element analysis and other methods). *Ann N Y Acad Sci*. 2006;1085:22–28.
161. White RA, Donayre C, Walot I et al. Abdominal aortic aneurysm rupture following endoluminal graft deployment: report of a predictable event. *J Endovasc Ther*. 2000;7:257–262.
162. Abraham CZ, Chuter TA, Reilly LM et al. Abdominal aortic aneurysm repair with Zenith stent graft: short to midterm results. *J Vasc Surg*. 2002;36:2117–2224.
163. Greenhalgh RM et al. Comparison of endovascular aneurysm repair with open repair in patients with abdominal aortic aneurysm (EVAR trial 1), 30-day operative mortality results: randomized controlled trial. *Lancet*. 2004; 364:843–848.
164. Blankensteijn JD et al. Two-year outcomes after conventional or endovascular repair of abdominal aortic aneurysms. *N Engl J Med*. 2005;352:2398–2405.
165. Carpenter JP et al. Durability of benefits of endovascular versus conventional abdominal aortic repair. *J Vasc Surg*. 2002;35:222–228.
166. Chahwan S et al. Elective treatment of abdominal aortic aneurysm with endovascular or open repair: the first decade. *J Vasc Surg*. 2007;45:258–262.
167. Goueffic Y et al. Midterm survival after endovascular versus open repair of infrarenal aortic aneurysms. *J Endovasc Ther*. 2005;12:47–57.
168. Brewster DC et al. Long-term outcomes after endovascular abdominal aortic aneurysm repair: the first decade. *Ann Surg*. 2006;244(3):426–438.

169. Lee WA et al. Perioperative outcomes after open and endovascular repair of intact abdominal aortic aneurysm in the United States during 2001. *J Vasc Surg*. 2004;39:491–496.

170. Moore WS et al. Five-year interim comparison of Guidant bifurcated endograft with open repair of abdominal aortic aneurysm. *J Vasc Surg*. 2003;38:46–55.

171. Elkouri S et al. Perioperative complications and early outcome after endovascular and open surgical repair of abdominal aortic aneurysms. *J Vasc Surg*. 2004;39:497–505.

172. Mani k, Bjork M, LUndkvist J. Improved long-term survival after abdominal aortic aneurysm repair. *Circulation*. 2009; 120(3):188–189.

173. Veith FJ, Lachat M, Mayer D et al. Collected world and single center experience with endovascular treatment of ruptured abdominal aortic aneurysms. *Ann Surg*. 2009;250: 818–824.

174. Lederle FA, Freischlag JA, Kyriakides TC et al. Outcomes following endovascular vs open repair of abdominal aortic aneurysms: a randomized trial. *JAMA*. 2009;302:1535–1542.

175. Krupski WC, Selzman CH, Floridia R et al. Contemporary management of isolated iliac artery aneurysms. *J Vasc Surg*. 1998;28:1–11.

176. Kasirajan V, Hertzer NR, Beven EG et al. Management of isolated common iliac artery aneurysms. *Cardiovasc Surg*. 1998;6:171–177.

177. Hirsch AT et al. ACC/AHA 2005 Guidelines for the management of patients with peripheral arterial disease (lower extremity, renal, mesenteric, and abdominal aortic): a collaborative report from the American Association for Vascular Surgery/Society for Vascular Surgery, Society for Cardiovascular Angiography and Interventions, Society for Vascular Medicine and Biology, Society of Interventional Radiology, and the ACC/AHA Task Force on Practice Guidelines (writing committee to develop guidelines for the management of patients with peripheral arterial disease). *J Am Coll Cardiol*. 2006;47:1–92.

178. Rajagopalan S, Mukherjee D et al. *Manual of Vascular Diseases*. Philadelphia: Lippincott Williams and Wilkins; 2005.

179. Hallett JW Jr. Splenic artery aneruysms. *Semin Vasc Surg*. 1995;8:321–326. 177.

180. Kasirajan K, Greenberg RK, Clair D et al. Endovascular management of visceral artery aneurysms. *J Endovasc Ther*. 2001;8:150–155.

181. Moore SW, Lewis RJ. Splenic artery aneurysm. *Ann Surg*. 1961;153(6):1033–1045.

182. Berceli S. Hepatic and Splenic artery aneurysms. *Semin Vasc Surg*. 2003; 18(4):196–201.

183. Stone WM, Abbas M, Cherry KJ et al. Superior mesenteric artery aneurysms: is presence an indication for intervention? *J Vasc Surg*. 2002;36:234–237.

184. Stone WM, Abbas MA et al. Celiac artery aneurysms: a critical reappraisal of a rare entity. *Arch Surg*. 2002;137:670–674.

185. Fisher DF Jr, Fry WJ. Collateral mesenteric circulation. *Surg Gynecol Obstet*. 1987;164:487–492.

186. Ottinger LW, Austin WG. A study of 136 patients with mesenteric infarction. *Surg Gynecol Obstet*. 1967;124:251–261.

187. Hertzer NR, Beven EG, Humphries AW. Acute intestinal ischemia. *Am Surg*. 1978;44:744–749.

188. Bergan JJ. Recognition and treatment of intestinal ischemia. *Surg Clin N Am*. 1967;47:109–126.

189. Jarvinen O, Laurikka J, Sisto T et al. Atherosclerosis of the visceral arteries. *Vasa*. 1995;24(1):9–14.

190. Wolf EA Jr, Sumner DS, Strandness DE Jr. Disease of the mesenteric circulation in patients with thromboangiitis obliterans. *Vasc Surg*. 1972;6:218–223.

191. Hollier LH, Bernatz PE, Pairolero PC et al. Surgical Management of chronic intestinal ischemia: a reappraisal. *Surgery*. 1981;90:940–946.

192. Johnston KW, Lindsay TF, Walker PM et al. Mesenteric arterial bypass grafts: early and late results and suggested surgical approach for chronic and acute mesenteric ischemia. *Surgery*. 1995;118:1–7.

193. Dunbar JD, Molnar W, Beman FF, Marable SA. Compression of the celiac trunk and abdominal angina: preliminary report of 15 cases. *AJR Am J Roentgenol*. 1966;95:731–744.

194. Reilly LM, Ammar AD, Stoney RJ, Ehrenfeld WK. Late results following operative repair for celiac artery compression syndrome. *J Vasc Surg*. 1985;2:79–91.

195. Vivian S et al. Celiac artery compression by the median arcuate ligament: a pitfall of end-expiratory MR imaging. *Radiology*. 2003;228:437–442.

196. Reuter SR. Accentuation of celiac compression by the median arcuate ligament of the diaphragm during deep expiration. *Radiology*. 1971;98:561–564.

197. Reuter SR, Bernstein EF. The anatomic basis for respiratory variation in median arcuate ligament compression of the celiac artery. *Surgery*. 1973;73:381–385.

198. Rajagopalan S, Mukherjee D et al. *Manual of Vascular Diseases*. Philadelphia: Lippincott Williams and Wilkins; 2005.

199. Abud O, Chechile GE, Lole-Balcells F. Aneurysm and arteriovenous malformation. In: Novick AC, Scoble JE, Hamilton G, eds. *Renal Vascular Disease*. London, UK: WB Saunders; 1996:35–46.

200. Novick AC. Renal artery aneurysms and arteriovenous malformations. In: Novick AC, Straffon RA, eds. *Vascular Problems in Urologic Surgery*. Philadelphia, PA: WB Saunders; 1982:189–204.

201. Hansen KJ, Edwards MS, Craven TE et al. Prevalence of renovascular disease in the elderly: a population-based study. *J Vasc Surg*. 2002;26:443–451.

202. Harding MB, Smith LR, Himmelstein SI et al. Renal artery stenosis: prevalence and associated risk factors in patients undergoing routine cardiac catheterization. *J Am Soc Nephrol*. 1992;2:1608–1616.

203. Weber-Mzell D, Kotanko P, Schumacher M et al. Coronary anatomy predicts presence or absence of renal artery stenosis: a prospective study in patients undergoing cardiac catheterization for suspected coronary artery disease. *Eur Heart J*. 2002;23:1684–1691.

204. Choudhri AH, Cleland JG, Rowlands PC et al. Unsuspected renal artery stenosis in peripheral vascular disease. *BMJ*. 1990;301:1197–1198.

205. Swartbol P, Thorvinger BO, Parsson H et al. Renal artery stenosis in patients with peripheral vascular disease and its correlation to hypertension: a retrospective study. *Int Angiol*. 1992;11:195–199.

206. Missouris CG, Papavassiliou MB, Khaw K et al. High prevalence of carotid artery disease in patients with atheromatous renal artery stenosis. *Nephrol Dial Transplant*. 1998;13: 945–948.

207. Balk EM et al. Comparative effectiveness of management strategies for renal artery stenosis. Comparative effectiveness review No. 5. Prepared by Tufts-New England Medical Center Evidence-based Practice Center under Contract No. 2900-02-0022. Agency for Healthcare Research and Quality; October 2006; Rockville, MD. Available at: www.effective-healthcare.ahrq.gov/reports/final.cfm.

208. Leertouwer TC, Pattynama PM, van den Berg-Huysmans A. Incidental renal artery stenosis in peripheral vascular diseasease: a case for treatment? *Kidney Int*. 2001;59:1480–1483.

209. Luscher TF, Keller HM, Imhof HG et al. Fibromuscular hyperplasia: extension of the disease and therapeutic outcome. results of the University Hospital Zurich Cooperative Study on fibromuscular hyperplasia. *Nephron*. 1986; 44(Suppl 1):109.

210. Mettinger KL. Fibromuscular dysplasia and the brain. II. Current concept of the disease. *Stroke*. 1982;13:53.

211. Estepa R, Gallego N, Orte L et al. Renovascular hypertension in children. *Scand J Urol Nephrol*. 2001;35:388.

212. Chiche L, Bahnini A, Koskas F, Kieffer E. Occlusive fibromuscular disease of arteries supplying the brain: results of surgical treatment. *Ann Vasc Surg*. 1997;11:496.

213. Slovut DP, Olin JW. Fibromuscular dysplasia. *N Engl J Med*. 2004; 350:1862.

214. Sauer L, Reilly LM, Goldstone J et al. Clinical spectrum of symptomatic external iliac fibromuscular dysplasia. *J Vasc Surg*. 1990;12:488.

215. Kolluri R, Ansel G. Fibromuscular dysplasia of bilateral brachial arteries–a case report and literature review. *Angiology*. 2004;55:685.

216. Begelman SM, Olin JW. Fibromuscular dysplasia. *Curr Opin Rheumatol*. 2000;12:41.

217. Stanley JC, Gewertz BL, Bove EL et al. Arterial fibrodysplasia. Histopathologic character and current etiologic concepts. *Arch Surg*. 1975;110:561.

218. Schievink WI, Bjornsson J. Fibromuscular dysplasia of the internal carotid artery: a clinicopathological study. *Clin Neuropathol*. 1996;15:2.

219. Luscher TF, Lie JT, Stanson AW et al. Arterial fibromuscular dysplasia. *Mayo Clin Proc*. 1987;62:931.

220. Dziewas R, Konrad C, Drager B et al. Cervical artery dissection–clinical features, risk factors, therapy and outcome in 126 patients. *J Neurol*. 2003;250:1179.

221. So EL, Toole JF, Dalal P, Moody DM. Cephalic fibromuscular dysplasia in 32 patients: clinical findings and radiologic features. *Arch Neurol*. 1981;38:619.

222. Mettinger KL, Ericson K. Fibromuscular dysplasia and the brain. I. Observations on angiographic, clinical and genetic characteristics. *Stroke*. 1982;13:46.

223. Honjo O, Yamada Y, Kuroko Y et al. Spontaneous dissection and rupture of common iliac artery in a patient with fibromuscular dysplasia: a case report and review of the literature on iliac artery dissections secondary to fibromuscular dysplasia. *J Vasc Surg*. 2004;40:1032.

224. Olin JW, Piedmonte M, Young JR et al. Utility of duplex scanning of the renal arteries for diagnosing significant renal artery stenosis. *Ann Intern Med*. 1995;122:833.

225. Vasbinder GB, Nelemans PJ, Kessels AG et al. Accuracy of computed tomographic angiography and magnetic resonance angiography for diagnosing renal artery stenosis. *Ann Intern Med*. 2004;141:674.

226. Gowda MS, Loeb AL, Crouse LJ, Kramer PH. Complementary roles of color-flow duplex imaging and intravascular ultrasound in the diagnosis of renal artery fibromuscular dysplasia: should renal arteriography serve as the "gold standard"? *J Am Coll Cardiol*. 2003;41:1305.

227. Carman T, Olin JW, Czum J. Noninvasive imaging of renal arteries. *Urol Clin N Am.* 2001;28:815.

228. Leung DA, Hoffmann U, Pfammatter T et al. Magnetic resonance angiography versus duplex sonography for diagnosing renovascular disease. *Hypertension.* 1999;33:726.

229. Kincaid OW, Davis GD, Hallermann FJ, Hunt JC. Fibromuscular dysplasia of the renal arteries. Arteriographic features, classification, and observations on natural history of the disease. *Am J Roentgenol Radium Ther Nucl Med.* 1968;104:271.

230. Schreiber MJ, Pohl MA, Novick AC. The natural history of atherosclerotic and fibrous renal artery disease. *Urol Clin N Am.* 1984;11:383.

231. Qanadli SD, Mesurolle B, Coggia M et al. Abdominal aortic aneurysm: pretherapy assessment with dual-slice helical CT angiography. *Am J Roentgenol.* 2000;174(1):181–187.

232. Romano M, Mainenti PP, Imbraiaco M et al. Mjultidetector row CT angiography of the abdominal aorta and lower extremities in patients with peripheral arterial occlusive disease: diagnostic accuracy and interobserver agreement. *Eur J Radiol.* 2004;50(3):303–308.

233. Theisen D, Von Tengg-Kobligk H, Michaely H et al. CT angiography of the aorta. *Radiologe.* 2007;47(11):982–992.

234. Furukawa A, Kanasaki S, Kono N et al. CT diagnosis of acute mesenteric ischemia from various causes. *Am J Roentgenol.* 2009;192:408–416.

235. Cademartiri F, Palumbo A, Maffei E et al. Noninvasive evaluation of the celiac trunk and superior mesenteric artery with multislice CT in patients with chronic mesenteric ischemia. *Radiol Med.* 2008;113:1135–1142.

236. Chernyak V, Rozenblit AM, Patlas M et al. Type II endoleak after endoaortic graft implantation: diagnosis with helical CT angiography. *Radiology.* 2006;240(3):885–893.

237. Stavropoulos SW, Clark TW, Carpenter JP et al. Use of CT angiography to classify endoleaks after endovascular repair of abdominal aortic aneurysms. *J Vasc Interv Radiol.* 2005;16(5):663–667.

238. Saba L, Pascalis L, Montisci R et al. Diagnostic sensitivity of multidetector-row spiral computed tomography angiography

in the evaluation of type-II endoleaks and their source: comparison between axial scans and reformatting techniques. *Acta Radiol.* 2008;49(6):630–637.

239. Willmann JK, Wildermuth S, Pfammatter T et al. Aortoiliac and renal arteries: prospective intraindividual comparison of contrast-enhanced three-dimensional MR angiogrpay and multi-detector row CT angiography. *Radiology.* 2003;226: 798–811.

240. Rountas C, Viychou M, Vassiou K et al. Imaging modalities for renal artery stenosis in suspected renovascular hypertension: prospective intraindividual comparison of color Doppler US, CT angiography, GD-enhanced MR angiography, and digital subtraction angiography. *Ren Fail.* 2007;29(3): 295–302.

241. Fraioli F, Catalano C, Bertoletti L et al. Multidetector-row CT angiography of renal artery stenosis in 50 consecutive patients: prospective interobserver comparison with DSA. *Radiol Med.* 2006;111(3):459–468.

242. Tank PW et al. *Grant's Dissector.* Hagerstwon, MD: Lippincott Williams & Wilkins; 2005:128.

243. Criqui MH, Denenberg JO, Langer RD et al. The epidemiology of peripheral arterial disease: importance of identifying the population at risk. *Vasc Med.* 1997;2:221–226.

244. Hiatt WR, Hoag S, Hamman RF. Effect of diagnostic criteria on the prevalence of peripheral arterial disease. The San Luis Valley Diabetes Study. *Circulation.* 1995;91(5):1472–1479.

245. Selvin E, Erlinger TP. Prevalence of and risk factors for peripheral arterial disease in the United States: results from the National Health and Nutrition Examination Survey, 1999–2000. *Circulation.* 2004;110(6):738–743.

246. Hirsch AT, Criqui MH, Treat-Jacobson D et al. Peripheral arterial disease detection, awareness, and treatment in primary care. *JAMA.* 2001;286:1317–1324.

247. Selvin E et al. Prevalence of and risk factors for peripheral arterial disease in the United States: results from the NHANES 1999–2000. *Circulation.* 2004;110:738–743.

248. Becker GJ et al. The importance of increasing public and physician awareness of peripheral arterial disease. *J Vasc Interv Radiol.* 2002;12(1):7–11.

249. Smith SC et al. Atherosclerotic vascular disease conference: writing Group II: risk factors. *Circulation*. 2004; 109:2613.

250. Murabito JM et al. Intermittent claudication. A risk profile from the Framingham Heart Study. *Circulation*. 1997;96:44.

251. Kannel WB, Skinner JJ, Schwartz MJ et al. Intermittent claudication: incidene in the Framingham Study. *Circulation*. 1970;41:875–883.

252. Selvin E, Marinopoulos S, Berkenblit G et al. Meta-analysis: glycosylated hemoglobin and cardiovascular disease in diabetes mellitus. *Ann Intern Med*. 2004;141(6):421–431.

253. Norgren L, Hiatt WR, Dormandy JA et al. Inter-society consensus for the management of peripheral arterial disease (TASC II). *J Vasc Surg*. 2007;45(1):S5–S67.

254. Jude EB et al. Peripheral Arterial disease in diabetic and nondiabetic patients: a comparison of severity and outcome. *Diab Care*. 2001;24:1433.

255. Criqui MH, Vargas V, Denenberg JO et al. Ethnicity and peripheral arterial disease: the San Diego Population Study. *Circulation*. 2005;112(17):2703–2707.

256. Meijer WT, Hoes AW, Rutgers D et al. Peripheral arterial disease in the elderly: the Rotterdam Study. *Arterioscler Thromb Vasc Biol*. 1998;18:185–192.

257. Hirsch AT et al. ACC/AHA 2005 Guidelines for the management of patients with peripheral arterial disease (lower extremity, renal, mesenteric, and abdominal aortic): a collaborative report from the American Association for Vascular Surgery/Society for Vascular Surgery, Society for Cardiovascular Angiography and Interventions, Society for Vascular Medicine and Biology, Society of Interventional Radiology, and the ACC/AHA Task Force on practice guidelines (writing committee to develop guidelines for the management of patients with peripheral arterial disease). *J Am Coll Cardiol*. 2006;47:1–92.

258. McDermott MM et al. Leg symptoms in peripheral arterial diseae: associated clinical characteristics and functional impairment. *JAMA*. 2001;286:1599.

259. Stewart K, Hiatt W, Regensteiner J et al. Exercise training for claudication. *N Engl J Med*. 2002;347(24):1941–1951.

260. Regensteiner J, Ware JJ, McCarthy W et al. Effect of cilostazol on treadmill walking, community –based walking ability,
and health-related quality of life in patients with intermittent
claudication due to peripheral arterial disease: meta-analysis
of six randomized controlled trials. *J Am Geriatr Soc*.
2002;50(12):1939–1946.
261. Girolami B, Bernardi E, Prins M et al. Pran-training, smoking cessation, pentoxifylline, or nafronyl: a meta-analysis.
Arch Intern Med. 1999;159(4):337–345.
262. Hood SC, Moher D, Barber GG. Management of intermittent claudicaiton with pentoxifylline: meta-analysis of randomized controlled trials. *CMAJ*. 1996;155(8):1053–1059.
263. Moher D, Pham B, Ausejo M et al. Pharmacological management of intermitten claudication: a meta-analysis of randomized trials. *Drugs*. 2000;59(5):1057–1070.
264. Beard JD. Which is the best revascularization for critical
limb ischemia: endovascular or open surgery? *J Vasc Surg*.
2008;48:11S–16S.
265. Stoeckelhuber BM, Meissner O, Stoeckelhuber M et al.
Primary endovascular stent placements of focal infrarenal
aortic stenosis. Initial and mid term results. *J Vasc Interv
Radiol*. 2003;14:1443–1447.
266. Simons PC, Nawijn AA, Bruijninkcx CM et al. Long-term
results of primary stent placement to treat infrarenal aortic
stenosis. *Eur J Vasc Endovasc Surg*. 2006;32:627–633.
267. Becker GJ, Katzen BT, Dake MD. Noncoronary angioplasty.
Radiology. 1989;170(3):921–940.
268. Rutherford R, Durham J. Percutaneous balloon angioplasty
for arteriosclerosis obliterans: long term results. In: Yao J,
Pearce W, eds. *Techniques in Vascular Surgery*. Philadelphia:
Saunders; 1992:329–345.
269. Murphy TP, Ariaratnam NS, Carney WI et al. Aortoiliac
insufficiency: long term experience with stent placement for
treatment. *Radiology*. 2004;231(1):243–249.
270. Timaran CH, Stevens SL, Freeman MB et al. External iliac
and common iliac artery angioplasty and stenting in men and
women. *J Vasc Surg*. 2001;34(3):440–446.
271. Tetteroo E, van der Graaf Y, Bosch JL et al. Randomized comparison of primary stent placement versus primary angioplasty followed by selective stent placement in patients with

iliac-artery occlusive disease. Dutch Iliac Stent Trial Study Group. *Lancet.* 1998;18(351):1153–1159.

272. Klein WM, van der Graaf Y, Seegers J et al. Long-term cardiovascular morbidity, mortality, and reintervention after endovascular treatment in patients with iliac artery disease: the Dutch Iliac Stent Trial Study. *Radiology.* 2004;232(2): 491–498.

273. Bosch JL, Hunink MG. Meta-analysis of the results of percutaneous transluminal angioplasty and stent placement for aortoiliac occlusive disease. *Radiology.* 1997;204(i): 87–96.

274. Ponec D, Jaff MR, Swischuk J et al. The NItinol SMART stent vs Wallstent for suboptimal iliac artery angioplasty: CRISP-US Trial results. *J Vasc Interv Radiol.* 2004; 15(9):911–918.

275. Wolf GL, Wilson SE, Cross AP et al. Surgery or balloon angioplasty for peripheral vascular disease; a randomized clinical trial. *J Vasc Interv Radiol.* 1993;4:639–648.

276. Kim YW, Lee JH, Kim HG et al. Factors affecting the long-term patency of crossover femorofemoral bypass graft. *Eur J Vasc Endovasc Surg.* 2005;30:376–380.

277. Ricco JB, Probst H. Long-term results of a multicenter randomized study on direct versus crossover bypass for unilateral iliac artery occlusive disease. *J Vasc Surg.* 2008; 47:45–53.

278. Sabeti S, Schillinger M, Amighi J et al. Primary patency of femoro-popliteal arteries treated with Nitonol stainless steel self expanding stents: propensity score adjusted analysis. *Radiology.* 2004;232:516–521.

279. Vogel TR, Shindelman LE, Nackman JB et al. Efficacious use of Nitinol stents in the femoral and popliteal arteries. *J Vasc Surg.* 2003;38:1178–1184.

280. Jahnke T, Voshage G, Muller-Hulsbeck S et al. Endovascular placement of self expanding Nitinol coiled stents for the treatment of femoropopliteal obstructive disease. *J Vasc Interv Radiol.* 2002;13:257–266.

281. Muradin G, Bosch J, Stijnen T et al. Balloon dilation and stent implantation for treatment of femoropopliteal arterial disease: meta-analysis. *Radiology.* 2001;221(1): 137–145.

282. Schillinger M, Sabeti S, Loewe C et al. Balloon angioplasty versus implantation of nitinol stents in the superficial femoral artery. *N Engl J Med*. 2006;354(18):1879–1888.

283. Duda SH, Bodier SM, Lammer J et al. Sirolimus eluting vs bare Nitinol stents for obstructive superficial fermoral artery disease. The SIROCCO II trial. *J Vasc Interv Radiol*. 2005;16:331–338.

284. Duda SH, Bosiers M, Lammer J et al. Drug-eluting and bare nitinol stents for the treatment of atherosclerotic lesions in the superficial femoral artery: long-term results from the SIROCCO trial. *J Endovasc Ther*. 2006;13: 701–710.

285. Zeller T, Rastan A, Sixt S et al. Long-term results after directional atherectomy of femoro-popliteal lesions. *J Am Coll Cardiol*. 2006;48:1573–1578.

286. Kandzari DE, Kiesz RS, Allie D et al. Procedural and clinical outcomes with catheter-based plaque excision ni critical limb ischemia. *J Endovasc Ther*. 2006;13:12–22.

287. Keeling WB, Shames ML, Stone PA et al. Plaque excision with the SilverHawk catheter: early results in patients with claudication or critical limb ischemia. *J Vasc Surg*. 2007;45:25–31.

288. Scheinert D, Laird JR, Schroder M et al. Excimer laser-assisted recanalization of long, chronic superficial femoral artery occlusions. *J Endovasc Ther*. 2001;8:156–166.

289. Bosiers M, Peeters P, Elst FV et al. Excimer laser assister angioplasty ofr critical limb ischemia: results of the LACI Belgium study. *Eur J Vasc Endovasc Surg*. 2005;29: 613–619.

290. Stoner MC, deFreitas DJ, Phade SV et al. Mid-term results with laser atherectomy in the treatment of infrainguinal occlusive disease. *J Vasc Surg*. 2007;46:289–295.

291. Lipitz EC, Ohki T, Veith FJ et al. Does subintimal angioplasty have a role in the treatment of severe lower extremity ischemia? *J Vasc Surg*. 2003;37:386–439.

292. Lazaris AM, Tsiamis AC, Fishwick G et al. Clinical outcome of primary infrainguinal subintimal angioplasty in

diabetic pateitns with critical lower limb ischemia. *J Endovasc Ther.* 2004;11:447–453.

293. Hynes N, Akhtar Y, Manning B et al. Subintimal angioplasty as a primary modality in the management of critical limb isehemia: comparison to bypass grafting for aortoiliac and femoropopliteal occlusive disease. *J Endovasc Ther.* 2004;11:460–471.

294. Schmieder GC, Panneton JM. Endovascular superficial femoral artery treatment: can it be as good as bypass? *Semin Vasc Surg.* 2008;21:186–194.

295. Laird J, Jaff MR, Biamino G et al. Cryoplasty for the treatment of femoropopliteal arterial disease: results of a prospective, multicenter registry. *J Vasc Interv Radiol.* 2005; 16:1067–1073.

296. Engelke C, Morgan RA, Belli AM. Cutting balloon percutaneous transluminal angioplasty for salvage of lower limb arterial bypass grafts: feasibility. *Radiology.* 2002;223: 106–114.

297. Bull PG, Mendel H, Hold M et al. Distal popoliteal and tibioperonealtransluminal angioplasty: long-term follow-up. *J Vasc Interv Radiol.* 1992;3:45–53.

298. Wolf G, Wilson S, Cross A et al. Surgery or balloon angioplasty ofr peripheral vascular disease: a randomized clinical trial. Principal investigators and their Associates of Veterans Administration Coooperative Study Number 199. *J Vasc Interv Radiol.* 1993;4(5):639–648.

299. Adam AJ, Beard JD, Cleveland T et al. BASIL trial participants. Bypass versus angioplasty in severe ischaemia of the leg (BASIL): multicenter, randomized controlled trial. *Lancet.* 2005;366:1925–1934.

300. Griffiths GD, Nagy J, Black D et al. Randomized clinical trial of distal anastemotic interposition vein cuff in infrainguinal polytetrafluoroethylene bypass grafting. *Br J Surg.* 2004;91:560–562.

301. Veith FJ, Gupta Sk, Ascer E et al. Six-year prospective multicenter randomized comparison of autologous saphenous vein and expanded polytetrafluoroethylene grafts in infrainguinal arterial reconstructions. *J Vasc Surg.* 1986;3:104–114.

302. Lam E, Landry G, Edwards J et al. Risk factors for autogenous infrainguinal bypass occlusion in patients with prosthetic inflow grafts. *J Vasc Surg*. 2004;39:336–342.

303. Albers M, Battistella V, Romiti M et al. Meta-analysis of polytetrafluoehtylene bypass grafts to infrapopliteal arteries. *J Vasc Surg*. 2003;37:1263–1269.

304. Jackson MR, Belott TP, Dickason T et al. The consequences of a failed femoropopliteal bypass grafting: comparison of saphenous vein and PTFE grafts. *J Vasc Surg*. 2000;32(3): 498–505.

305. London N, Srinivasan R, Naylor A et al. Subintimal angioplasty of femoropopliteal artery occlusions: the long-term results. *Eur J Vasc Surg*. 1994;8(2):148–155.

306. Abbott J, Williams D. Percutaneous treatment of peripheral arterial chronic total occlusions: device options and clinical outcomes. *Vasc Dis Manage*. 2007; 4. Available at: http://vasculardiseasemanagement.com/article/7540.

307. Desgranges P, Boufi M, Lapeyre M et al. Subintimal angioplasty: feasible and furable. *Eur J Vasc Endovasc Surg*. 2004;28(2):138–141.

308. Mossop P, Cincotta M, Whitbourn R. First case reports of controlled blunt microdissection for percutaneous transluminal angioplasty of chronic total occlusions in peripheral arteries. *Catheter Cardiovasc Interv*. 2003;59:255–258.

309. Aburahma AF, Robinson PA, Cook CC et al. Selecting patients for combined femoraofemoral bypass grafting and iliac balloon angioplasty and stenting for bilateral iliac disease. *J Vasc Surg*. 2001;33(2 suppl):S93–S99.

310. Hertzer NR, Bena JF, Karafa MT. A personal experience with direct reconstructionand extra-anatomic bypass for aortoiliofemoral occlusive disease. *J Vasc Surg*. 2007;45: 527–535.

311. Witness CH, van Houtte HJ, Van Urk H. European prospective randomized multi-center axillo-bifermoral tiral. *Eur J Vasc Surg*. 1992;6:115–123.

312. Smith FB, Lee AJ, Fowekes FG et al. Variation in cardiovascular risk factors by angiographic site of lower limb atherosclerosis. *Eur J Vasc Endovasc Surg*. 1996;11:340–346.

313. Scotland RS, Vallance PJ, Ahluwalia A. Endogenous factors involved in regulation of tone and arterial vasa vasorum: impl.ications for conduit vessel physiology. *Cardiovasc Res.* 2000;46:403–411.

314. Radonic V, Koplic S, Giunio L et al. Popliteal artery entrapment syndrome: diagnosis and management, with report of three cases. *Tex Heart Inst J.* 2000;27(1):3–13.

315. Hai Z, Guangrui S, Yan Z et al. CT angiography and MRI in patients with popliteal artery entrapment syndrome. *Am J Roentgenol.* 2008;191:1760–1766.

316. Graham LM, Zelenock GB, Whitehouse WM Jr et al. Clinical significance of arteriosclerotic femoral artery aneurysms. *Arch Surg.* 1980;115:502–507.

317. Whitehouse WM Jr, Wakefield TW, Graham LM et al. Limb threatening potential of arteriosclerotic popliteal artery aneurysms. *Surgery.* 1983;93:694–699.

318. Fuster V et al. *Hurst's The Heart.* 11th ed. McGraw-Hill; 2004:631.

319. Jarrett F, Makaroun MS, Rhee RY et al. Superficial femoral artery aneurysms: an unusual entity? *J Vasc Surg.* 2002; 36:571–574.

320. Cutler BS, Darling RC. Surgical management of arteriosclerotic femoral aneurysms. *Surgery.* 1973;74:764–773.

321. Duffy ST, Colgan MP, Sultan S et al. Popliteal aneurysms: a 10-year experience. *Eur J Vasc Endovasc Surg.* 1998;16: 218–222.

322. Taurino M, Calisti A, Grossi R et al. Outcome after early treatment of popliteal artery aneurysms. *Int Angiol.* 1998;17:28–33.

323. Szilagyi DE et al. Popliteal arterial aneurysm. Their natural history and management. *Arch Surg.* 1981;116:724.

324. Kaviani A, O'Hara PJ. 6 Vascular system, 17 Repair of femoral and popliteal artery aneurysms. In: Dale DC, Federman DD, eds. *ACS Surgery Online.* New York: WebMD Inc;2000. Available at: http://www.acssurgery.com/

325. Ailawadi G et al. Current conceps in the pathogenesis of abdominal aortic aneurysm. *J Vasc Surg.* 2003;38:584.

326. Varga ZA et al. A multicenter study of popliteal aneurysm. Joint Vascular Research Group. *J Vasc Surg*. 1994;20:171.

327. Aulivola B et al. Popliteal artery aneurysms: a comparison of outcomes in elective versus emergent repair. *J Vasc Surg*. 2004;39:1171.

328. Vermilion BD et al. A review of one hundred forty-seven popliteal aneurysms with long-term follow-up. *Surgery*. 1981;90:1009.

329. Gifford RW Jr, Hines EA Jr, Janes JM. An analysis and follow-up study of one hundred popliteal aneurysms. *Surgery*. 1953;33:284–293.

330. Lowell RC, Gloviczki P, Hallett JW Jr et al. Popliteal artery aneurysms: the risk of nonoperative management. *Ann Vasc Surg*. 1994;8:14–23.

331. Siauw R et al. Endovascular repair of popliteal artery aneurysms: techniques, current evidence and recent experience. *ANZ J Surg*. 2006;76:505.

332. Roggo A, Brunner U, Ottinger LW et al. The continuing challenge of aneurysms of the popliteal artery. *Surg Gynecol Obstet*. 1993;177:565–572.

333. Antonello M et al. Open repair versus endovascular treatment for asymptomatic popliteal artery aneurysm: results of prospective randomized study. *J Vasc Surg*. 2005;42:185.

334. Visser K, Idu MM, Buth J et al. Duplex scan surveillance during the first year after infrainguinal autologous vein bypass grafting surery: costs and clinical outcomes compared with other surveillance programs. *J Vasc Surg*. 2001;33(1):123–130.

335. Davies AH, Hawdon AJ, Sydes MR et al. Is duplex surveillance of value after leg vein bypass grafting? Principal results of the Vein Graft Surveillance Randomised Trial (VGST). *Circulation*. 2005;112(13):1985–1991.

336. Jacobs TF, Wintersperger BJ, Becker CR. MDCT-imaging of peripheral arterial disease. *Semin Ultrasound CT MR*. 2004;25(2):145–155.

337. Ota H, Takase K, Igarashi K et al. MDCT compared with digital subtraction angiography for assessment of lower extremity arterial occlusive disease: importance of reviewing

cross-sectional images. *AJR Am J Roentgenol.* 2004; 182(1):201–209.

338. Martin ML, Tay KH, Flak B et al. Multidetector CT angiography of the aortoiliac system and the lower extremeties: a prospective comparison with digital subtraction angiography. *Am J Roentgenol.* 2003;180:1085–1091.

339. Willmann JK, Mayer D, Banyai M et al. Evaluation of peripheral arterial bypass rafts with multi-detector row CT angiography: comparison with duplex US and digital subtraction angiography. *Radiology.* 2003;229:465–474.

340. Ofer A, Nitecki SS, Linn S et al. Multidetector CT angiography of peripheral vascular disease: a prospective comparison with intraarterial digital subtraction angiography. *Am J Roentgenol.* 2003;180:719–724.

341. Rubin GD, Schmidt AJ, Logan LJ et al. Multi-detector row CT angiography of lower extremity arterial inflow and runoff: initial experience. *Radiology.* 2001;221:146–158.

342. Catalano C, Fraioli F, Laghi A et al. Infrarenal aortic and lower extremity arterial disease: diagnostic performance of multi-detector row CT angiography. *Radiology.* 2004;231: 555–563.

343. Romano M, Mainenti PP, Imbriaco M et al. Multidetector row CT angiography of the abdominal aorta and lower extremities in patients with peripheral arterial occlusive disease: diagnostic accuracy and interobserver agreement. *Eur J Radiol.* 2004;50(3):303–308.

344. Piccoli G, Gasparini D, Smania S et al. Multislice CT angiography I the assessment of peripheral aneurysms. *Radiol Med.* 2003;106(506):504–511.

345. Rieker O, Duber C. Prospective comparison of CT angiography of the legs with intraarterial digital subtraction angiography. *Am J Roentgenol.* 1996;166(2):269–276.

346. Lopera JE, Trimmer CK, Josephs SG et al. Multidetector CT angiography of intrainguinal arterial bypass. *Radiographics.* 2008;28:529–549.

347. Hiratzka L, Bakris G, Beckman J et al. 2010 ACCF/AHA/ AATS/ACR/ASA/SCA/SIR/STS/SVM Guidelines for the diagnosis and management of patients with thoracic aortic disease: Executive summary: a report of the American

College of Cardiology Foundation/American Heart Association Task Force on Practice Guidelines, American Association for Thoracic Surgery, American College of Radiology, American Stroke Association, Society of Cardiovascular Anesthesiologists, Society for Cardiovascular Angiography and Interventions, Society of Interventional Radiology, Society of Thoracic Surgeons and Society for Vascular Medicine. *Circulation.* 2010;121:15; R. Pelberg, W. Mazur. *Vasc CT Angiography Manual.* 2010. doi:10.1007/978-1-84996-260-5_6.

348. Stary HC, Chandler AB, Dinsmore RE et al. A definition of advanced types of atherosclerotic lesions and a histological classification of atherosclerosis. A report from the Committee on Vascular Lesions of the Council on Arteriosclerosis, American Heart Association. *Circulation.* 1995;92: 1355–1374.

349. Coady MA, Ikonomidis JS, Cheung AT et al. Surgical management of descending thoracic aortic disease: open and endovascular approaches. A scientific statement from the American Heart Association. *Circulation.* 2010;121: 2780–2804.

350. Kligerman S, Blum A, Abbara S. Persistent fifth aortic arch in a patient with a history of intrauterine thalidomide exposure. *J Cardiovasc Comput Tomogr.* 2009;3:412–414.

Index

M